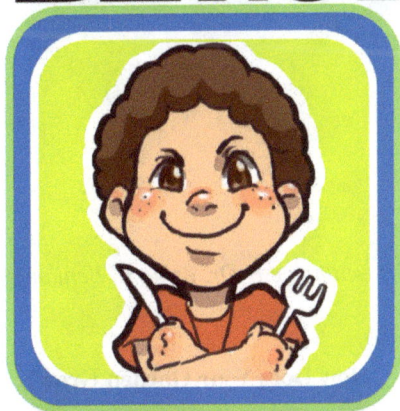

Healthy BENJI

How Does Your Garden Grow?

Dr. Benji's real name is Dr. Verna R. Benjamin-Lambert

How Does Your Garden Grow?

© 2012 by Dr. Verna R. Benjamin-Lambert

Library of Congress Control Number: 1817813

ISBN: 978-0-9910361-3-4

Printed in the United States of America

HOW DOES YOUR GARDEN GROW?

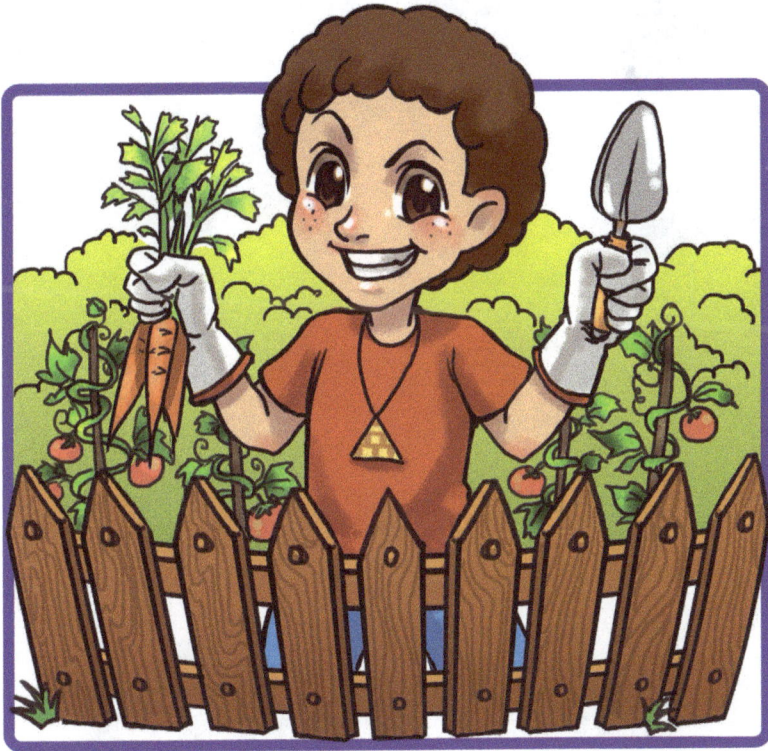

BY

DR. BENJI

ILLUSTRATED BY ARASHI YANG

HEALTHY READING FOR HEALTHY EATING!
BOOK FOR EARLY READERS

Health Intelligence, LLC.

To Parents and Teachers

The Healthy Benji book series brings excitement through reading about a variety of nutritious foods. Children will learn the value of various fruits and vegetables and understand how to make strategic choices as they nourish their bodies. The stories are designed to expose children to a wide array of food choices and for them to enjoy being a part of the preparation process.

Questions are asked at the end of each story to ensure that children understand and gain knowledge from what is read. Teachers and parents are encouraged to assist children in preparing meals using fresh fruits and vegetables to make dishes that children will find enjoyable to prepare and delicious to eat. When children become a part of the preparation process they will be more likely to try new things.

Throughout the Healthy Benji books series meaningful family connections are emphasized along with friendship, responsibility, manners, helpfulness, hygiene, appreciation and respect for others.

The Healthy Benji Book Series will help children develop healthy eating habits at a very early age. Through reading about and practicing healthy habits our children will have the best foundation possible to enjoy a wholesome and happy life.

LET'S START HERE! IT'S COOL TO BE HEALTHY

One afternoon, Healthy Benji went over to Ian's house to play. Ian showed Healthy Benji his vegetable garden.

"I want to grow a vegetable garden, too," said Healthy Benji.

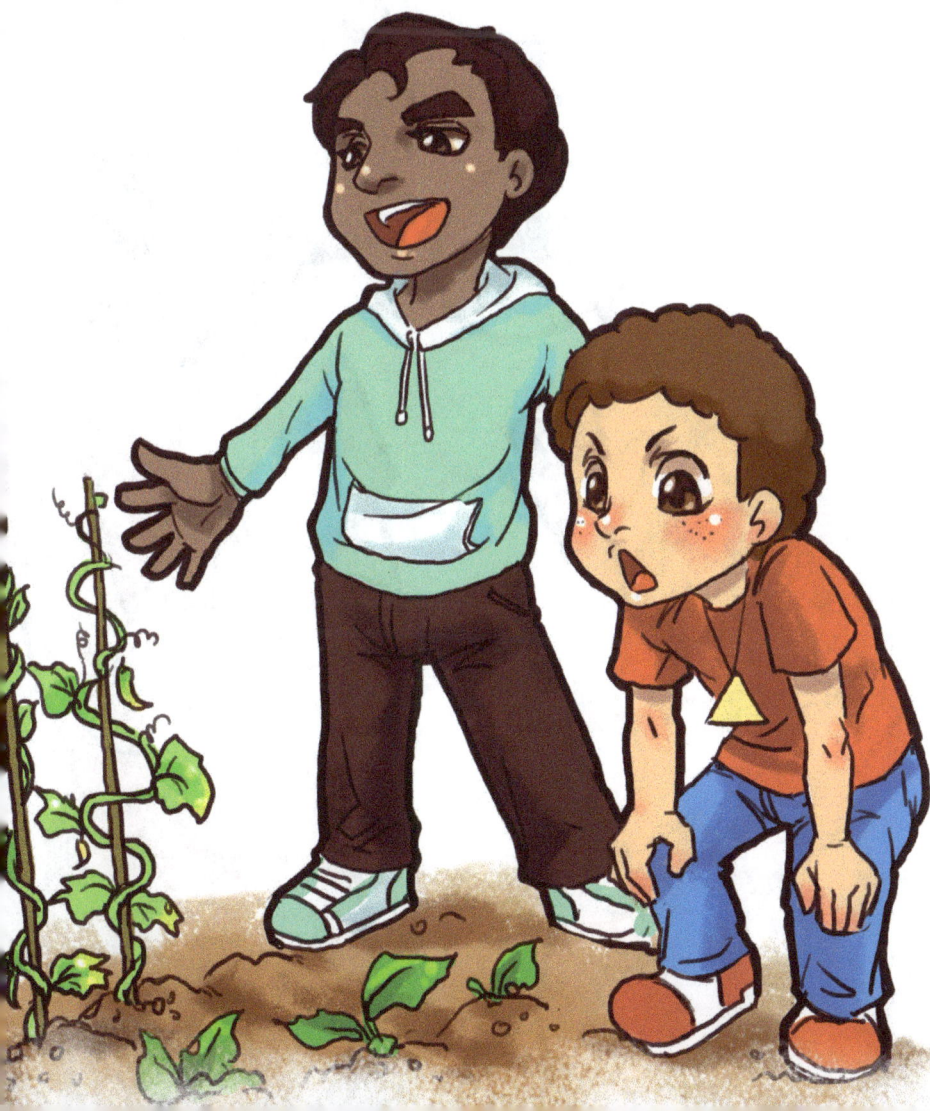

When he got home, Healthy Benji asked his mom if he could plant a vegetable garden. She was thrilled.

"Absolutely!" she said.

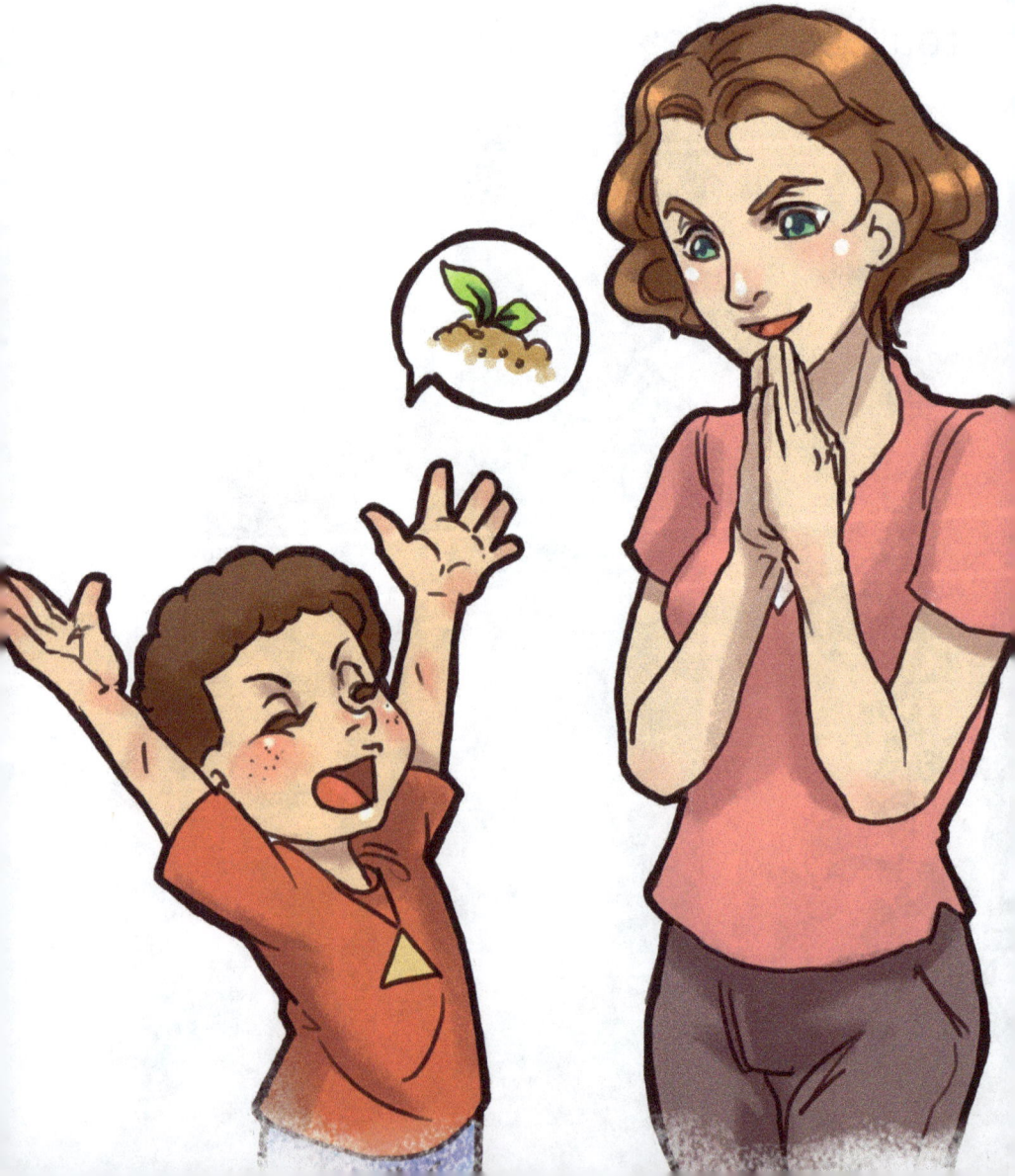

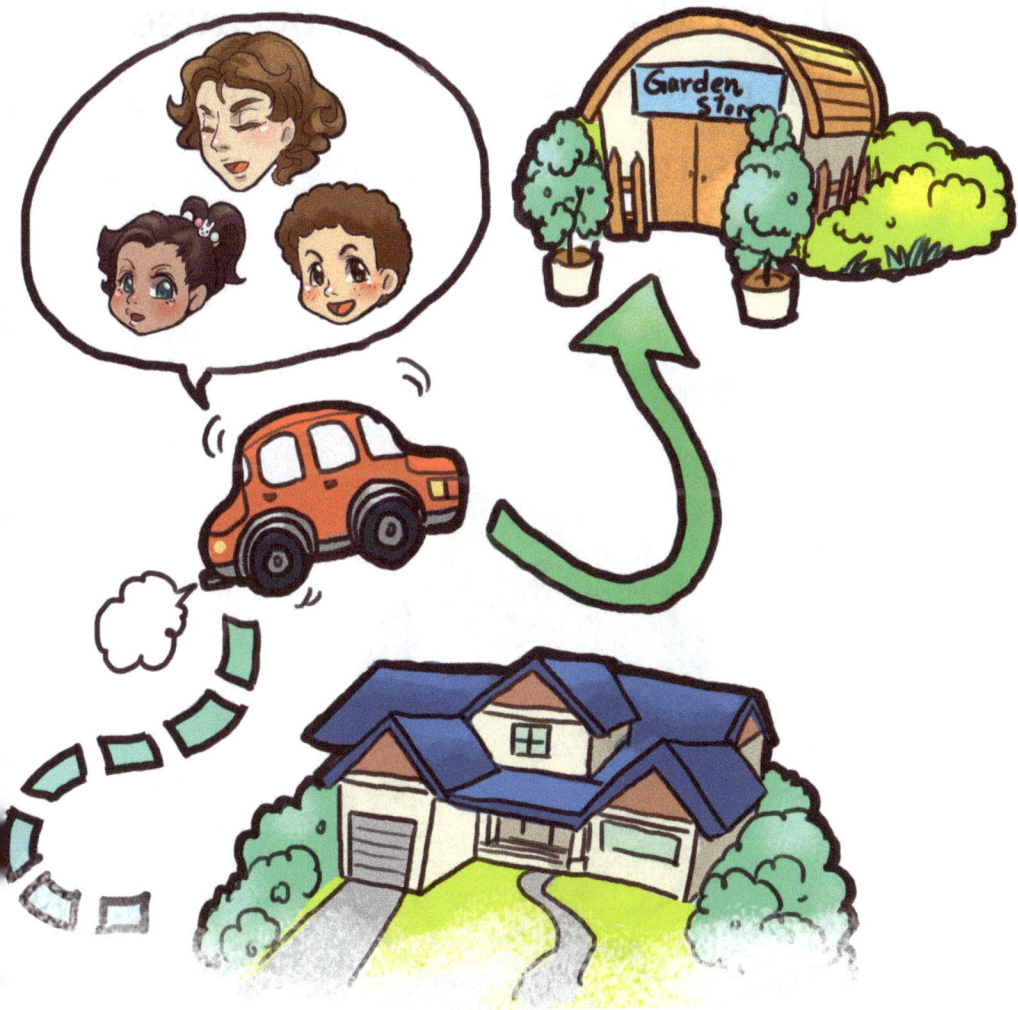

Nadia wanted to help. So, they took a trip to the home and garden store to shop for some vegetable seeds.

It was hard to decide because there were so many packets of seeds to choose from.

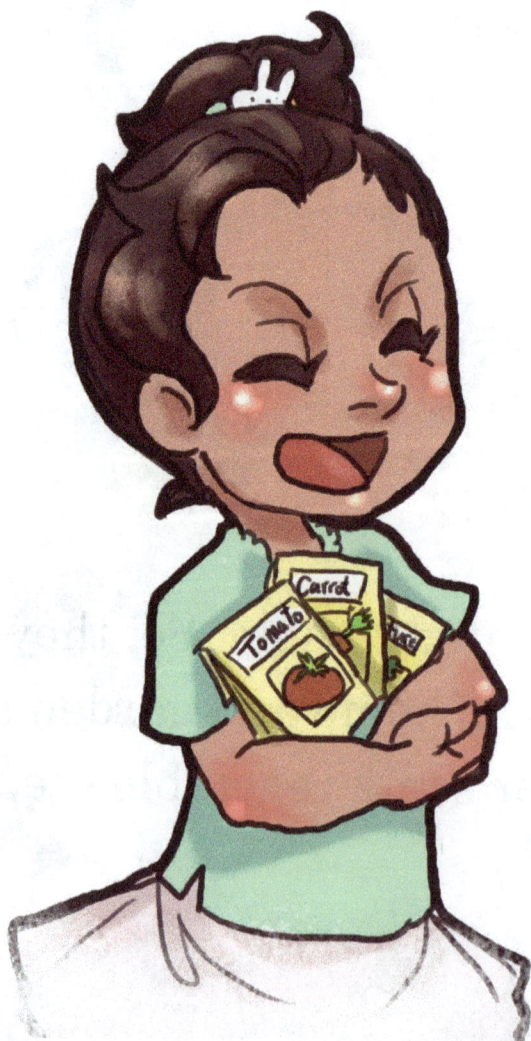

Healthy Benji chose zucchini, pumpkin, and green bean seeds. Nadia chose tomato, carrot, and lettuce seeds.

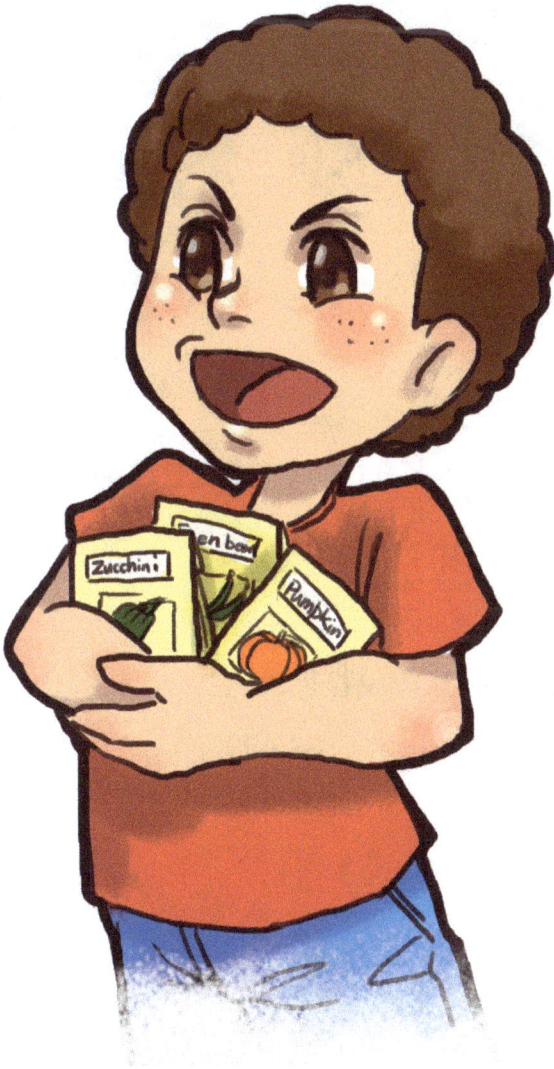

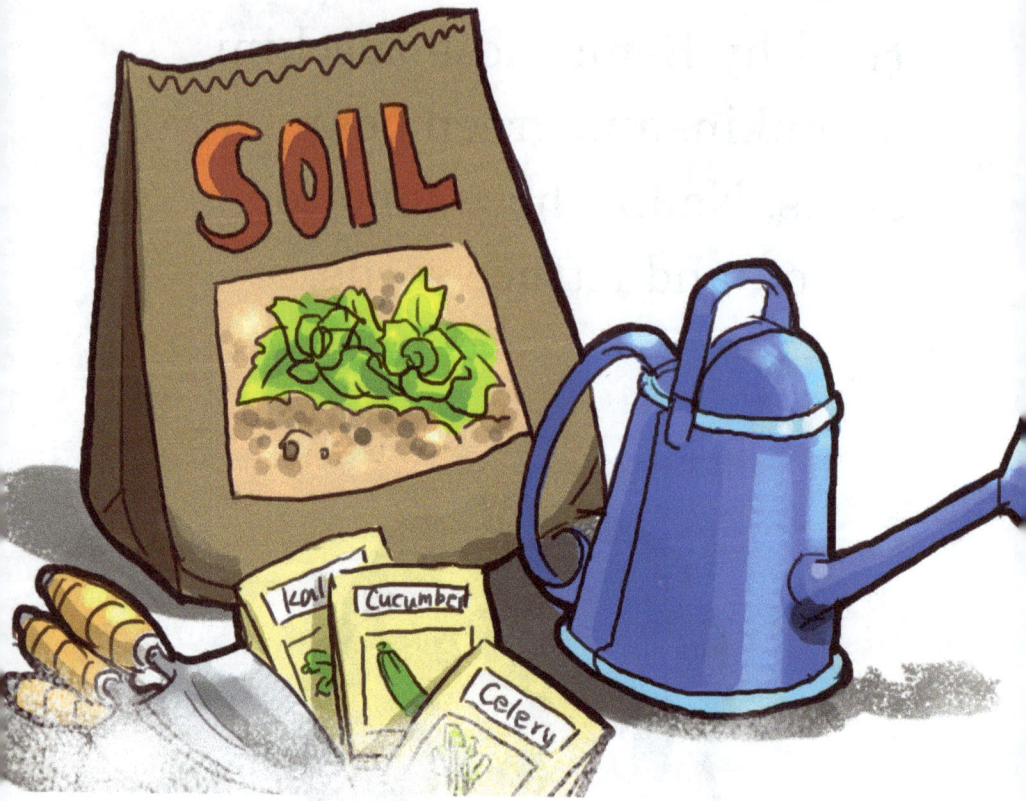

Mom chose kale, cucumber, and celery seeds.

They also bought soil, a watering can, and three small shovels.

When they got home, they blocked off a place in the backyard that would be just for the garden. Nadia put some wooden stakes in the ground, and Healthy Benji helped his mom put up a small fence to keep wild animals out of the garden.

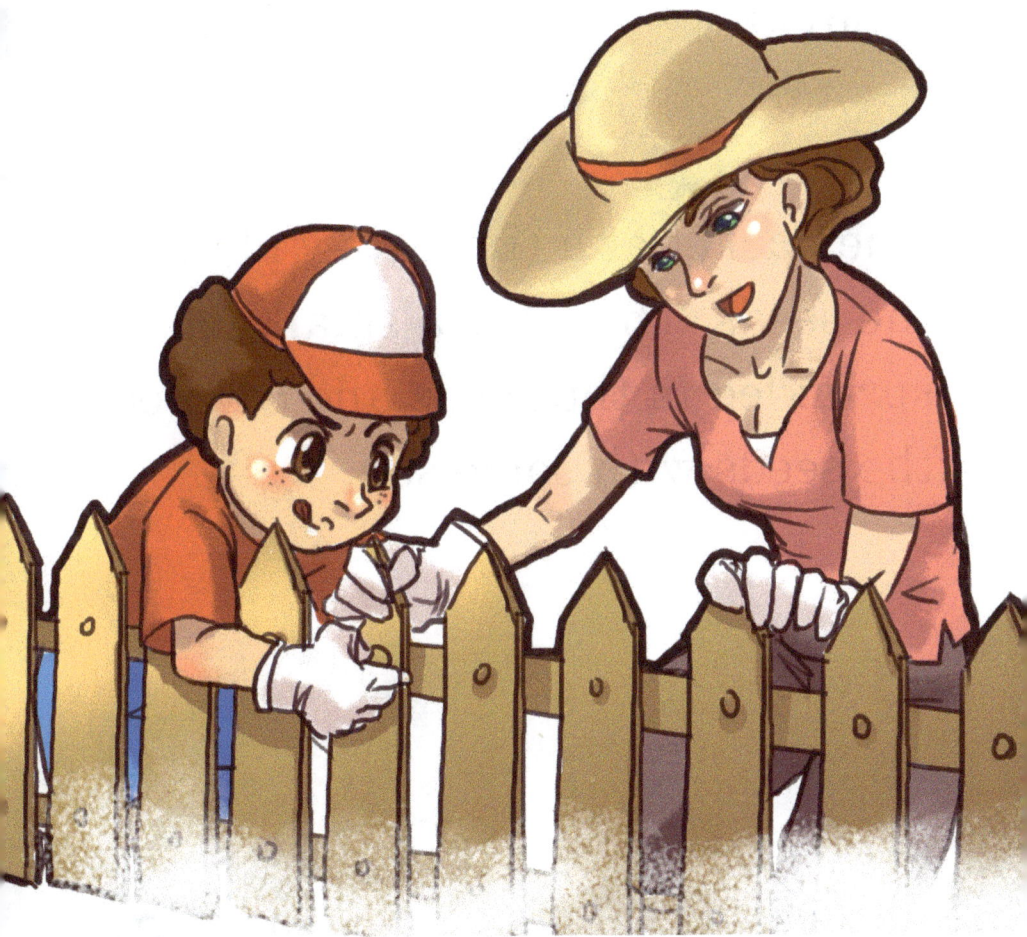

They read the directions on the back of each seed packet to make sure they knew how deep to plant the seeds and how far apart the seeds should be.

One packet at a time, they planted the seeds. They dug a small hole, sprinkled in the seeds and covered the seeds with some soil.

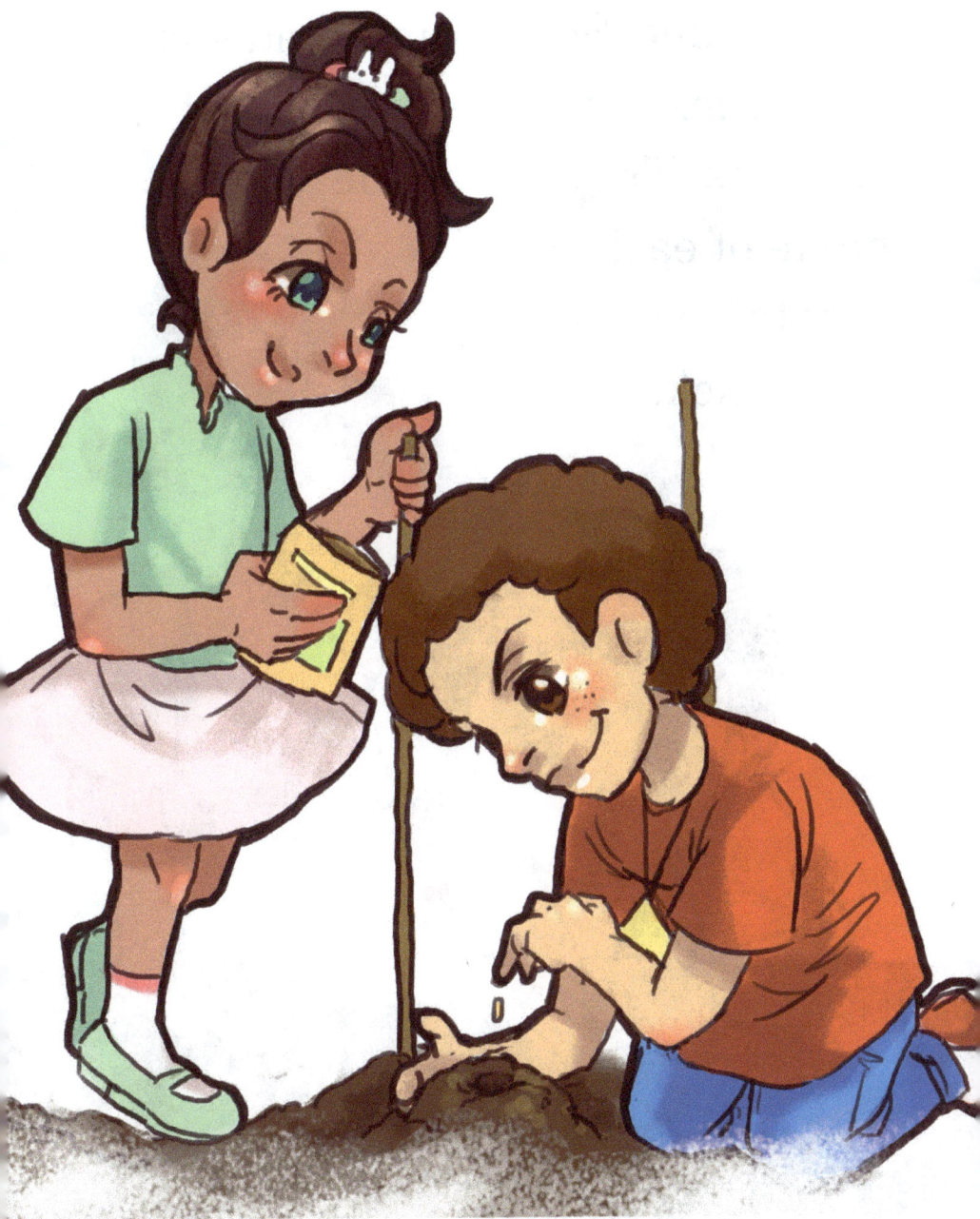

It's hard to remember what you've planted if you don't give yourself a reminder. So, Nadia found some craft sticks from her box of craft supplies. They wrote the name of each vegetable on a craft stick.

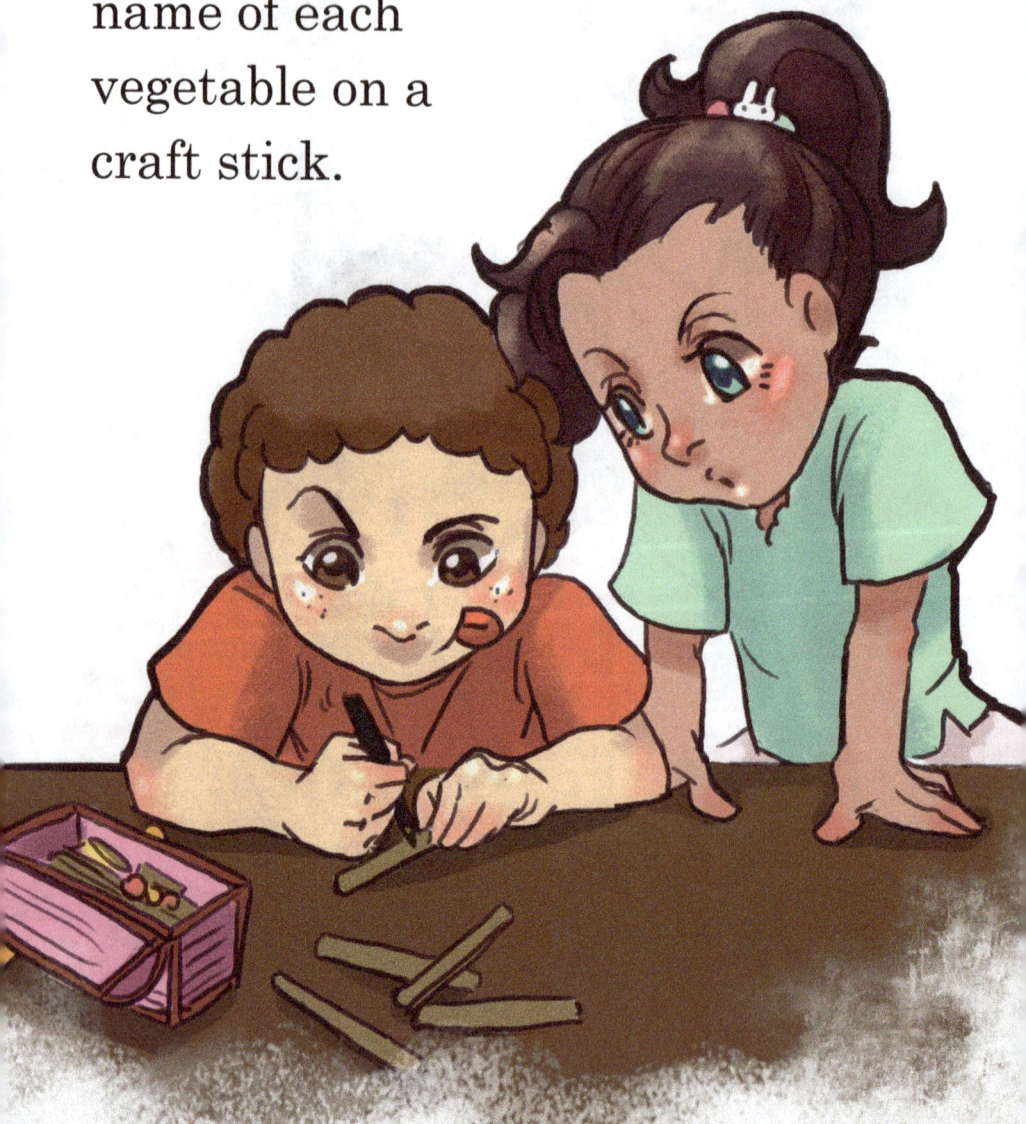

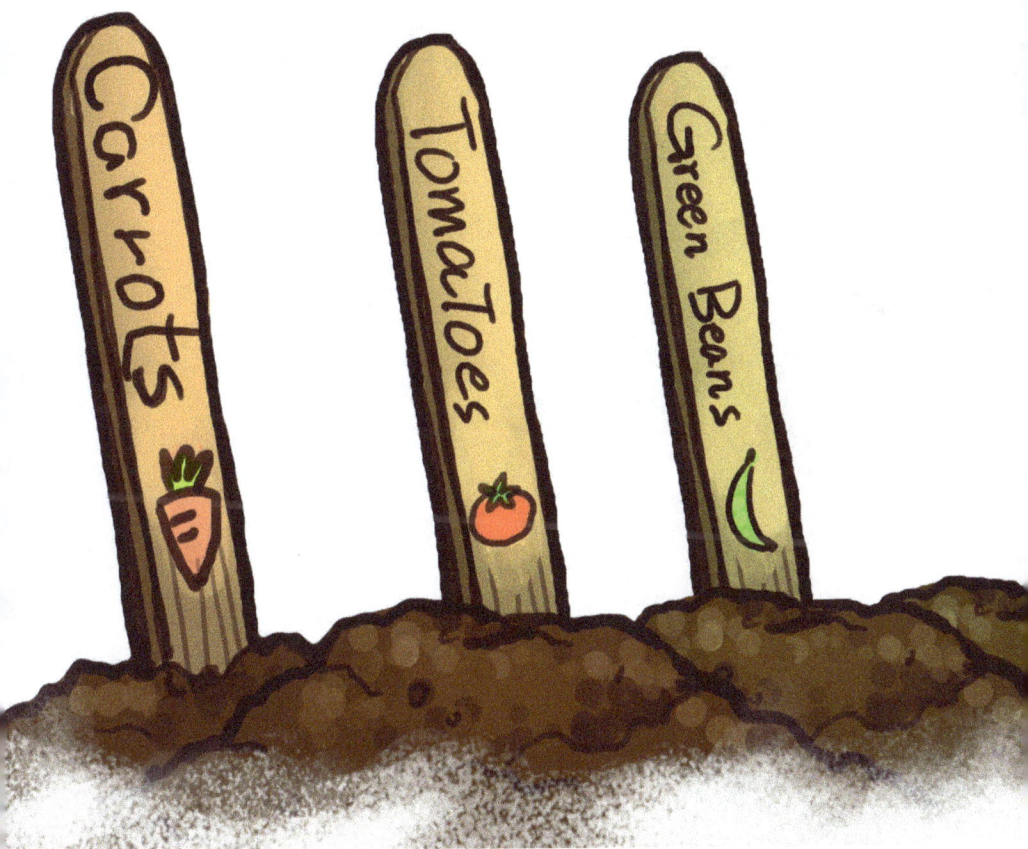

Then, they stuck the craft stick
label in the ground where they had
planted that vegetable. Perfect!
Now they would be able to tell what
vegetable was growing and where.

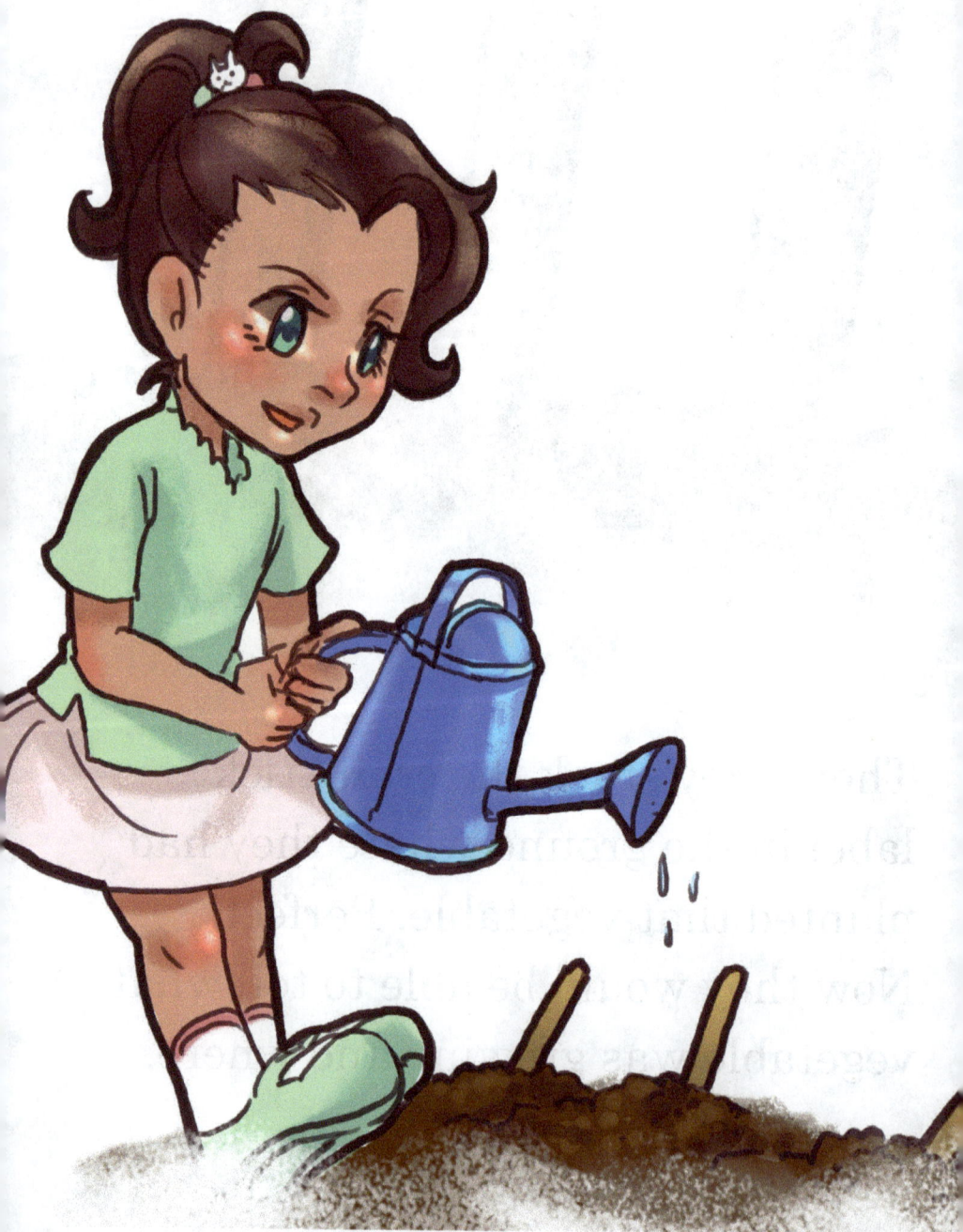

Soon, all the seeds had been planted. Nadia used the new watering can to gently water the seeds. Healthy Benji took a step back to check out the garden. "So, how long until we have vegetables?" asked Healthy Benji.

"Well," said his mom, "It's going to be a few weeks before we see any sprouts coming out of the ground." Healthy Benji made a funny face.

"I didn't know we'd have to wait that long," he said.

"Be patient, Healthy Benji. We'll check on the plants every day to see how they are growing," said Mom.

"Waiting is going to be hard," thought Healthy Benji.

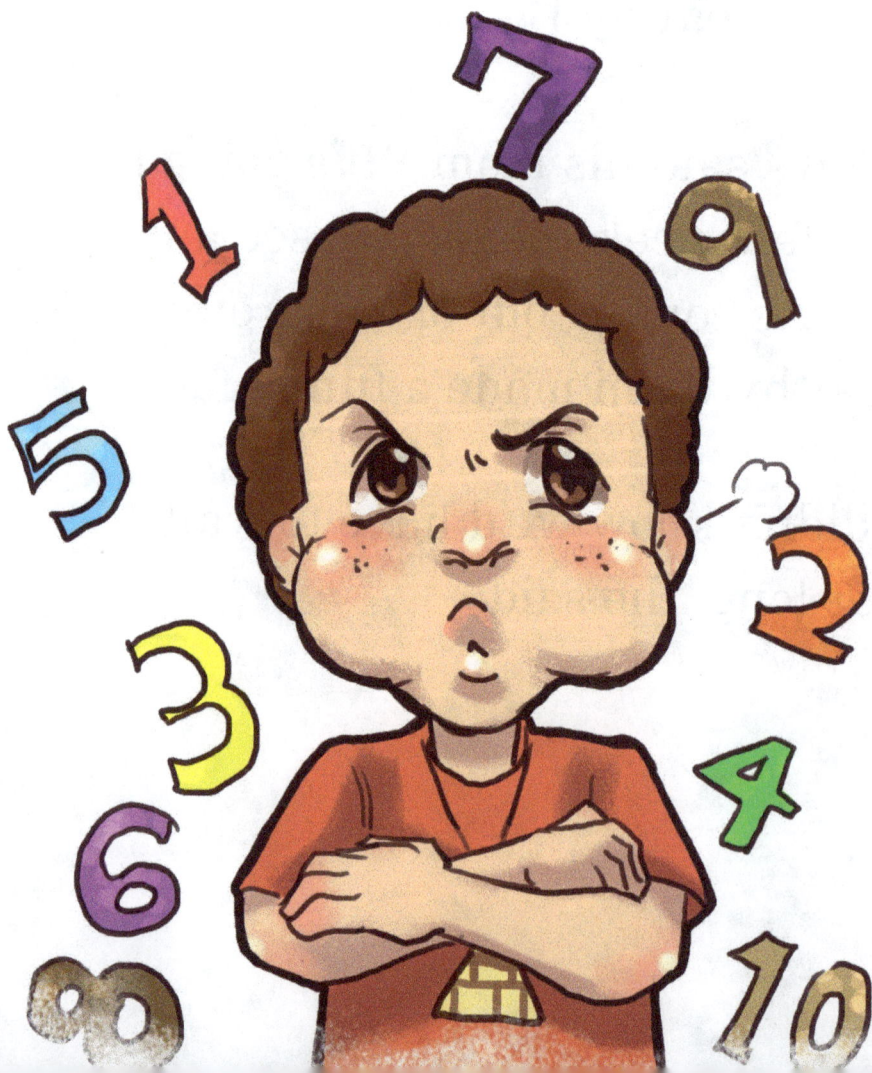

The next day, Healthy Benji checked on his garden. Nothing. "Bummer," he thought to himself. "Waiting is so hard," said Healthy Benji.

"It's only been one day," said Nadia.

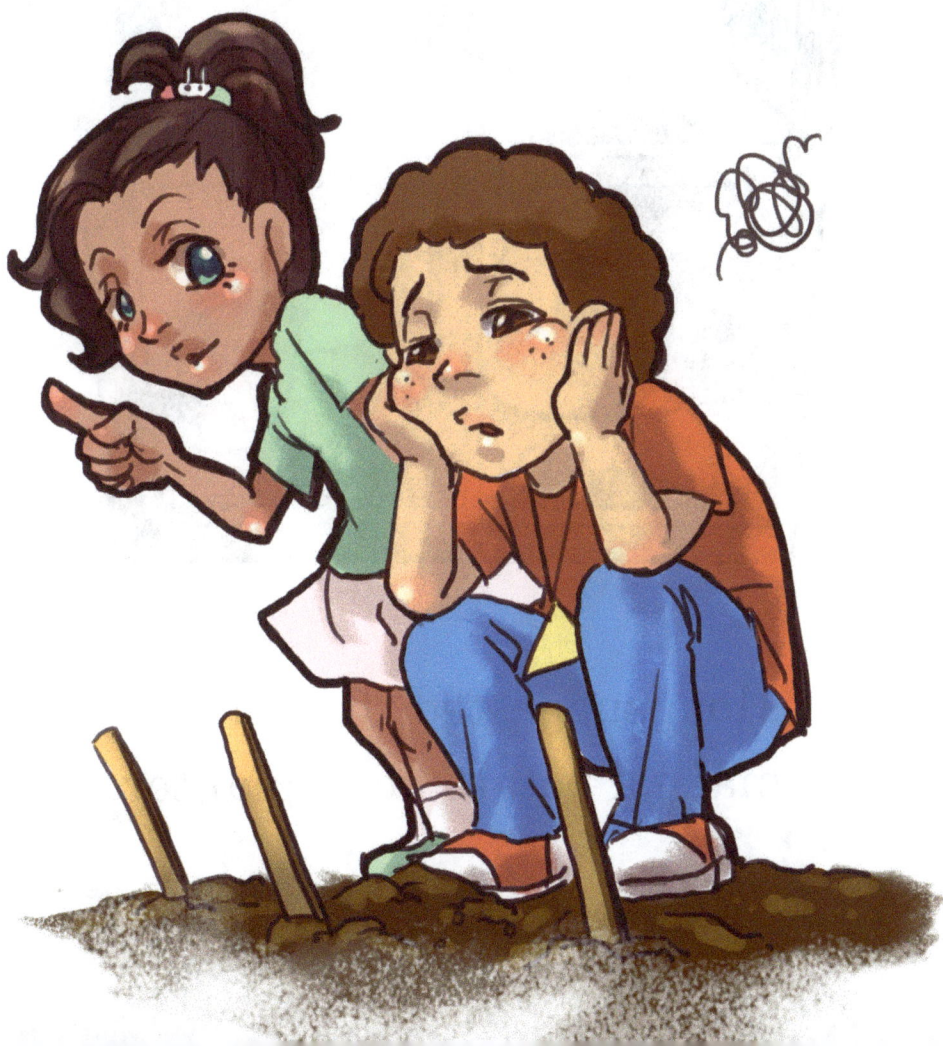

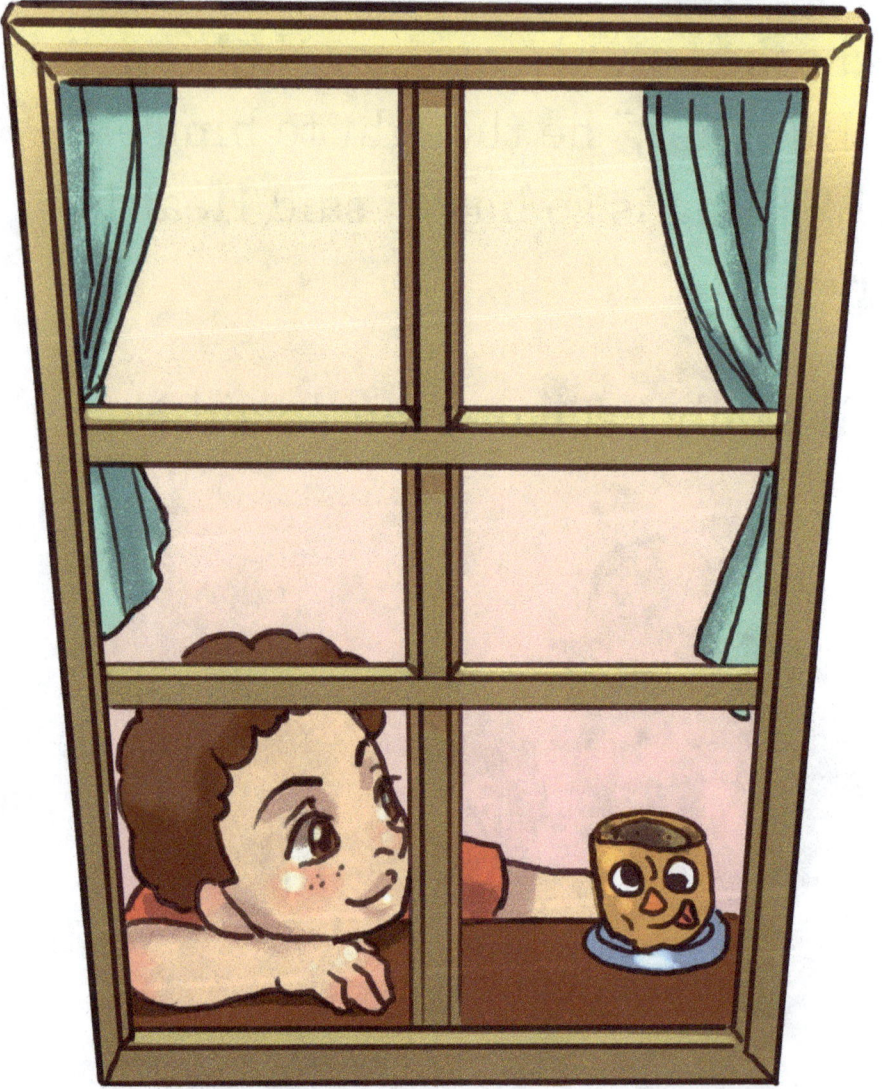

Mom suggested that they
make a potato head planter.

Healthy Benji started working on his planter and forgot all about waiting.

They took some cooked potatoes, scooped out the insides, put in some soil, added some grass seeds and covered them with more soil.

Healthy Benji made a a cute face on his potato head planter. They set them on the window sill so the seeds could get some sunlight.

In just a few days, Healthy Benji was so amazed to find that grassy hair was growing in his potato planter. It looked funny.

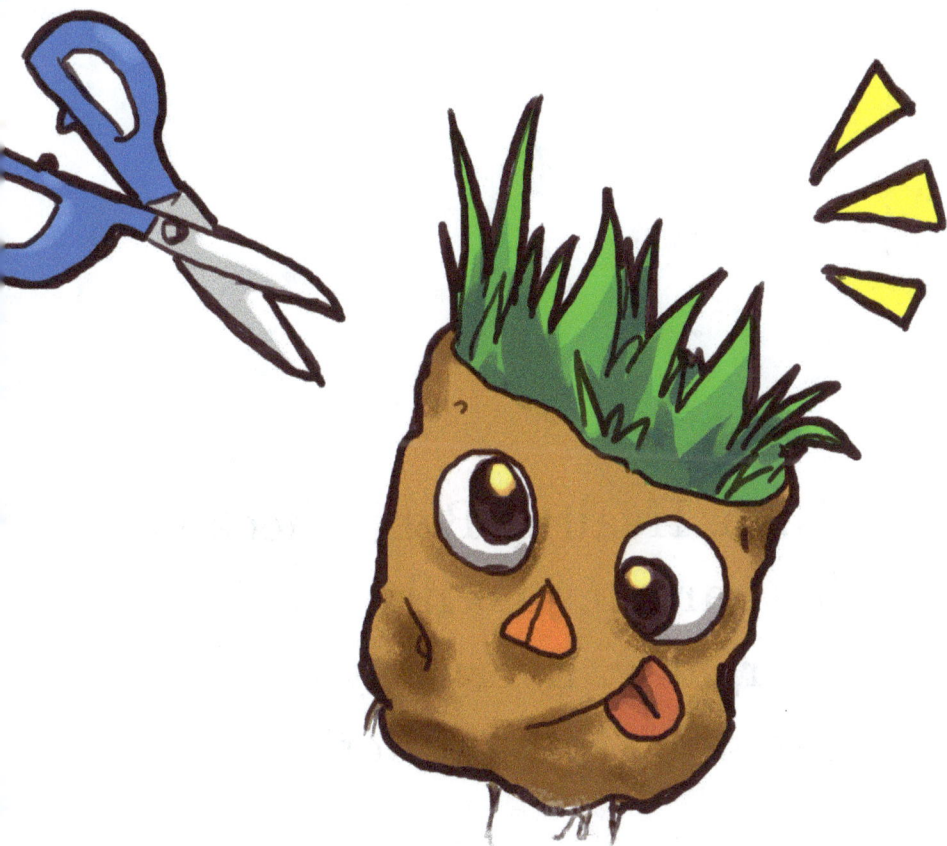

"That grew fast!" shouted Healthy Benji. "Yes," said Benji's mom, "Grass grows fast. That's why we have to cut our lawn at least once or twice a month"

Then, Healthy Benji checked his garden, just like he did every day. Every day it was the same thing – Nothing.

Until one day, Healthy Benji couldn't believe what he saw... sprouts! The plants were starting to grow! Healthy Benji was so excited!

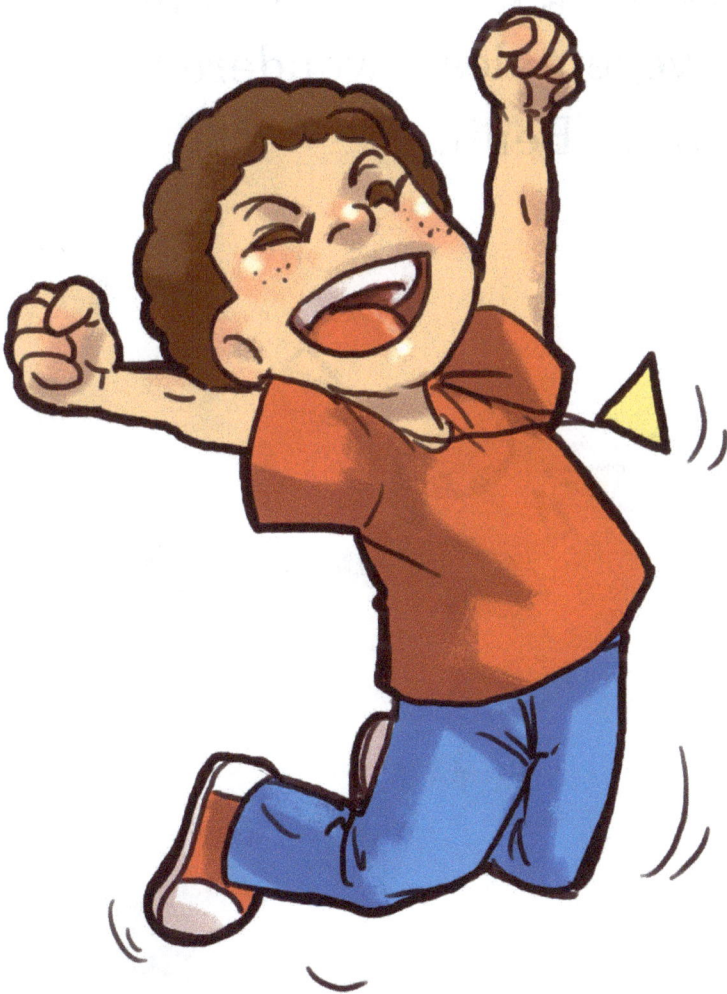

He ran to tell his mom and Nadia. They were excited, too.

"How long before we can pick the vegetables?" wondered Healthy Benji.

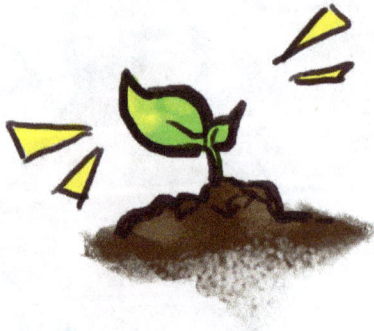

"They're just starting to grow," said Mom. They will need a few weeks to mature and grow.

"Ugh. A few weeks!?" Said Healthy Benji. "Oh, man. Waiting is hard!"

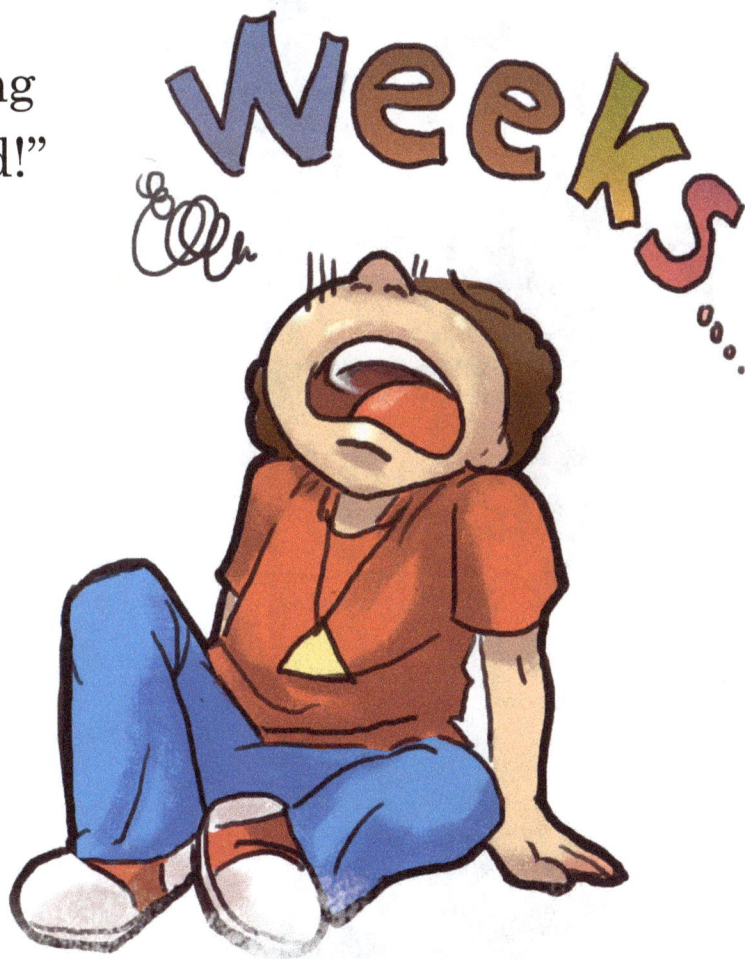

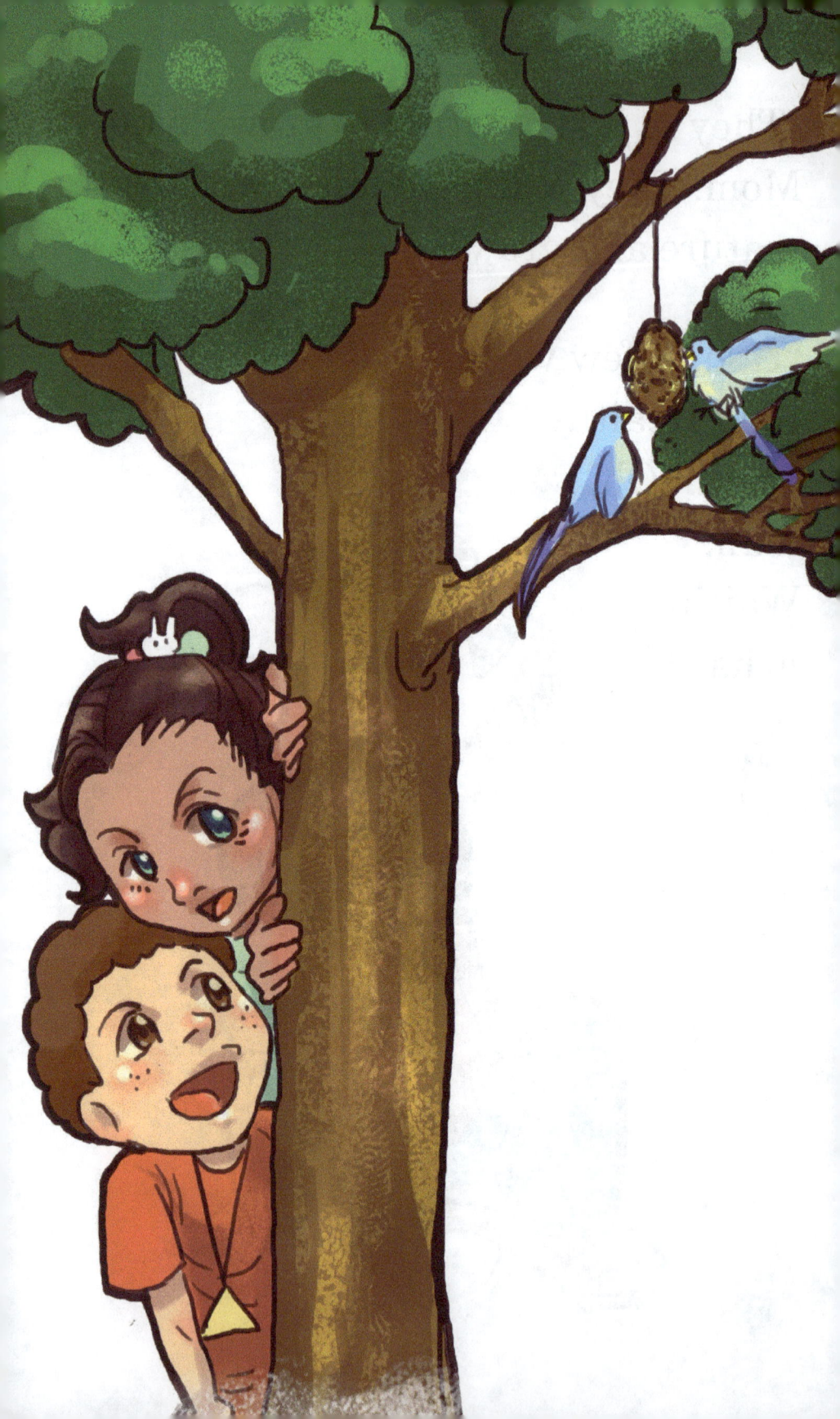

Benji's mom suggested they make a bird feeder. Once Healthy Benji started working on his bird feeder, he forgot all about waiting. He found a pinecone, slathered on some peanut butter, and rolled it in birdseed. Healthy Benji and Nadia hung the bird feeders in the trees for the birds. The birds loved them!

Healthy Benji kept checking the garden every day. He watered the plants. He watched. He waited. He growled, "This is taking too long". "

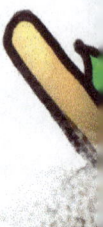

Be patient, Benji," said his mom,
"The plants are growing. They
just need more time."

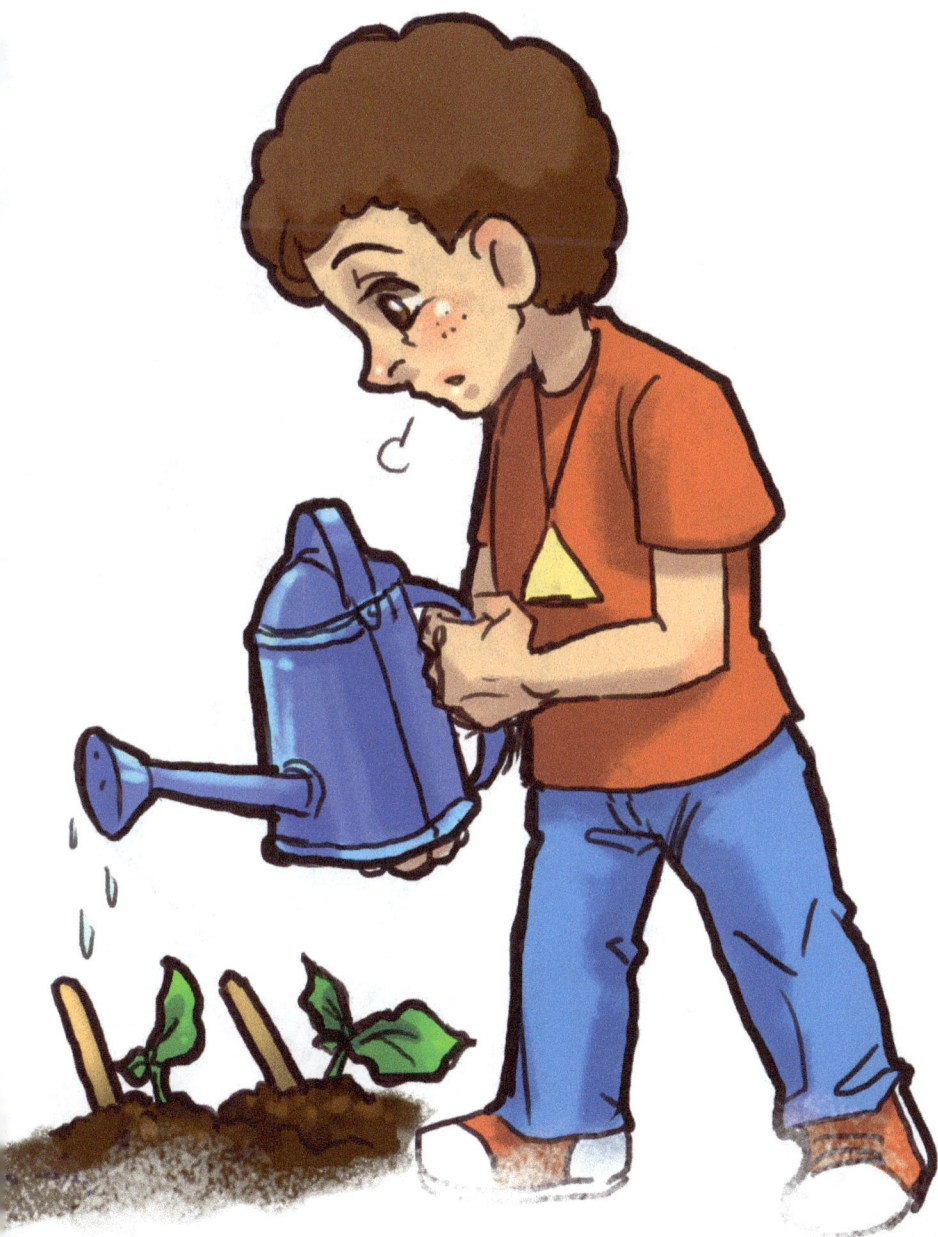

Benji's mom came up with another idea to keep his mind off the garden. She suggested that he feed the squirrels.

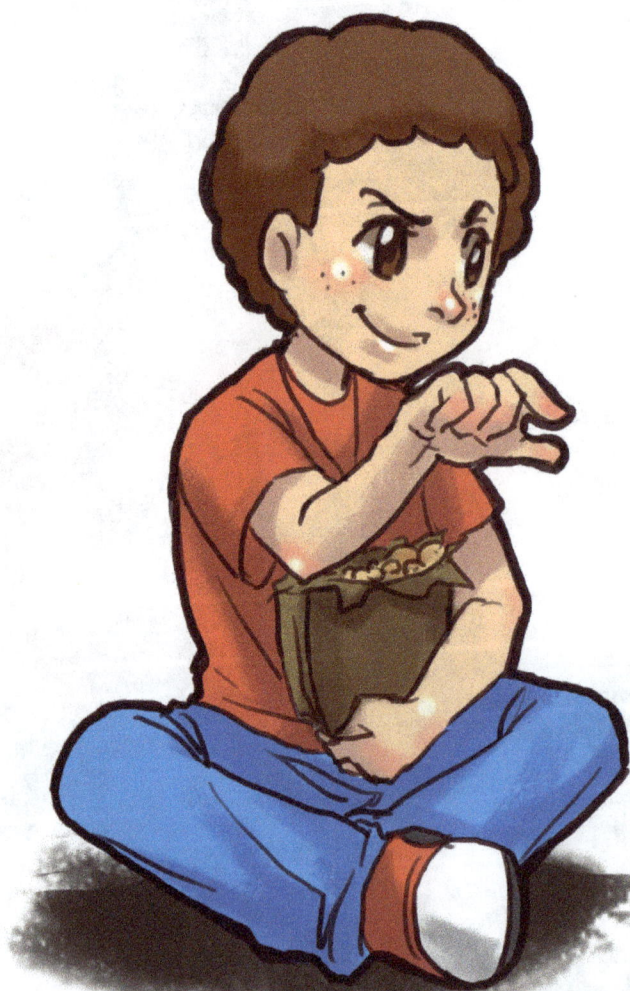

She gave Healthy Benji a large bag of peanuts, and off he went to find some squirrels.

Once he started throwing peanuts, he forgot all about waiting.
The squirrels were glad to keep Healthy Benji busy. They loved peanuts!

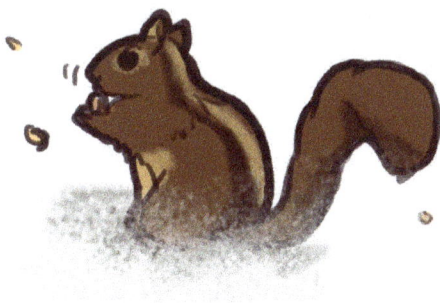

Then, one day, Healthy Benji checked his garden. "At last! At last!" He shouted. The plants looked terrific! They were growing taller, and vegetables were sprouting off the plants! They, actually, looked like vegetables. "Are they ready now?" Healthy Benji asked his mom.

"Almost," she said. Healthy Benji couldn't believe it. "More waiting? Ugh," he mumbled.

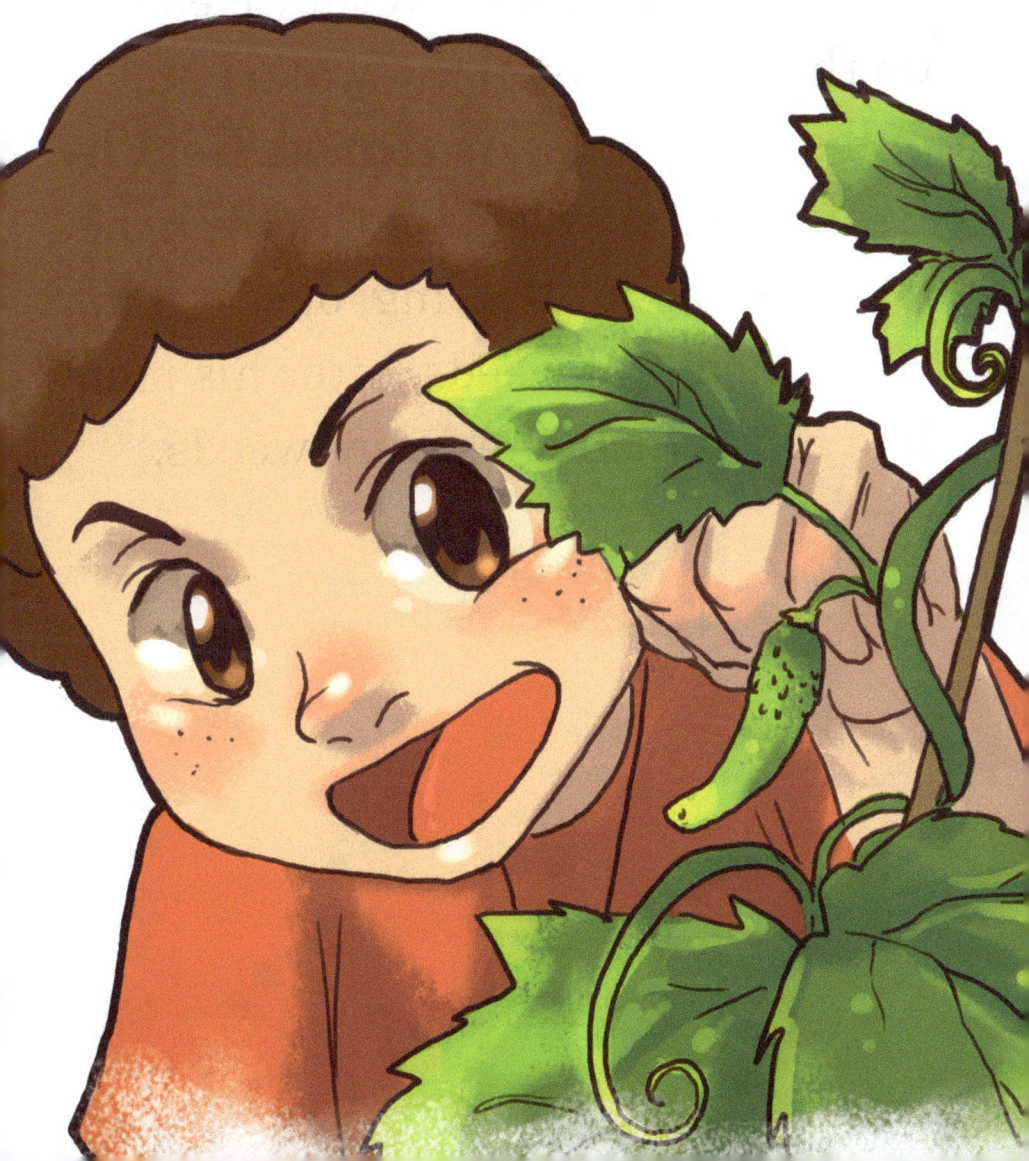

Benji's mom suggested they clean up the yard, sweep the walks, and pull some weeds. As soon as Healthy Benji started sweeping the walk, he forgot all about waiting, once again. He helped pull weeds, after his mom told him which ones were weeds.

He also found a few pieces of trash in the yard and put them in the garbage can.

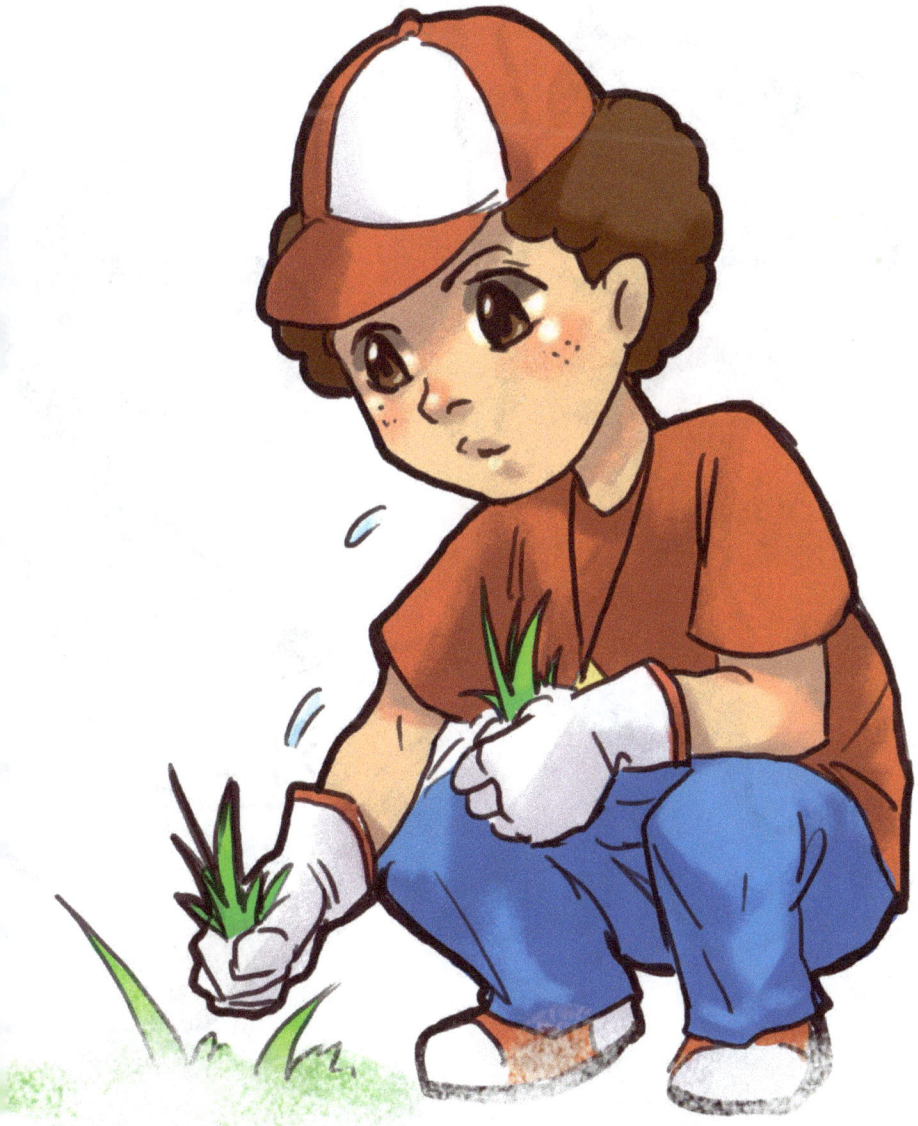

The next day, Benji's mom said,
"Benji, I think it's time to pick some
vegetables."

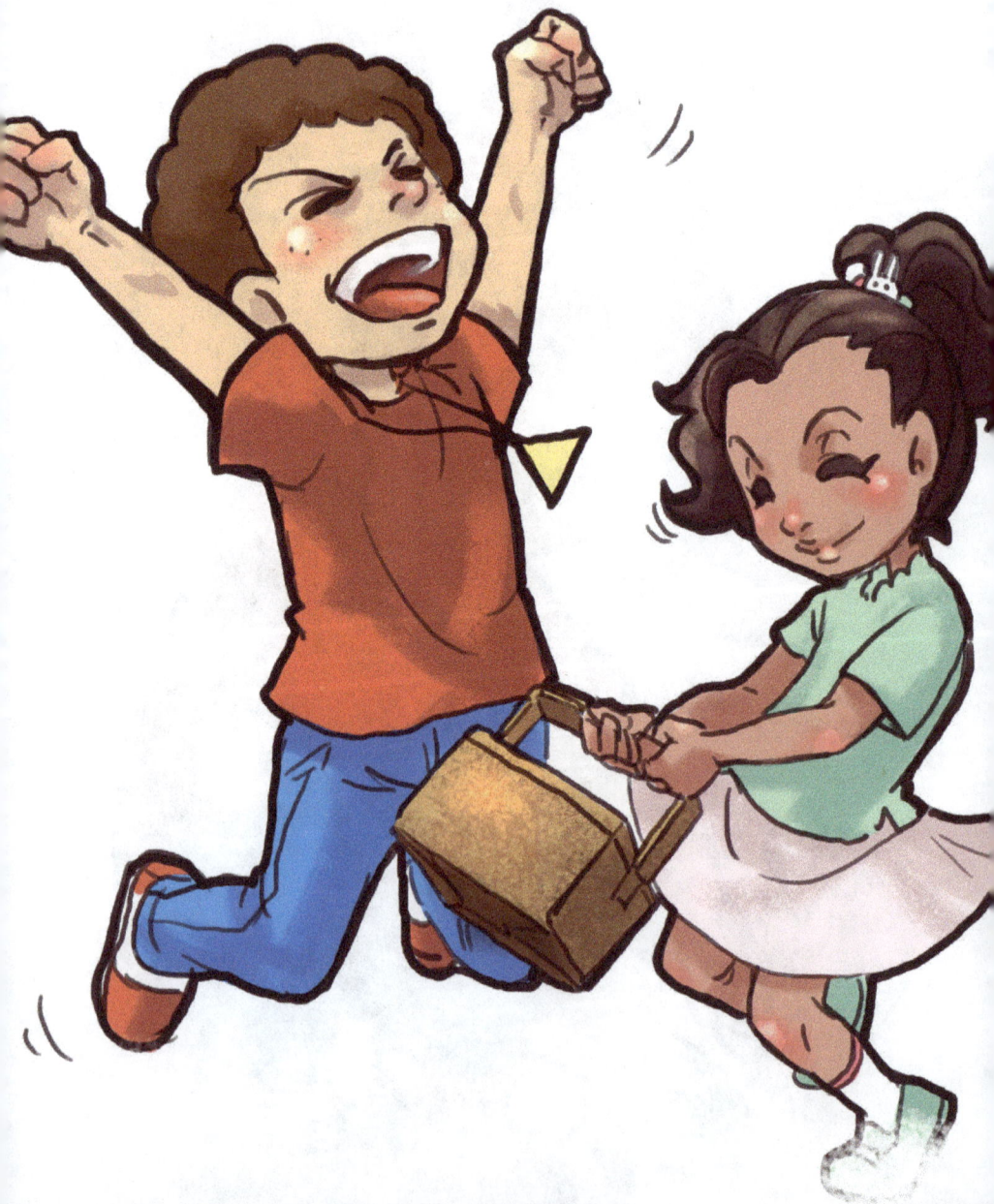

Healthy Benji was super excited. Nadia was very happy too. They went out to their garden and found they had grown – ready to be picked!

Healthy Benji, Nadia, and their mom picked zucchini, squash, green beans, tomatoes, and more. Everything looked so yummy! They took the vegetables inside and rinsed them with water. Healthy Benji and Nadia couldn't wait to taste what they'd grown.

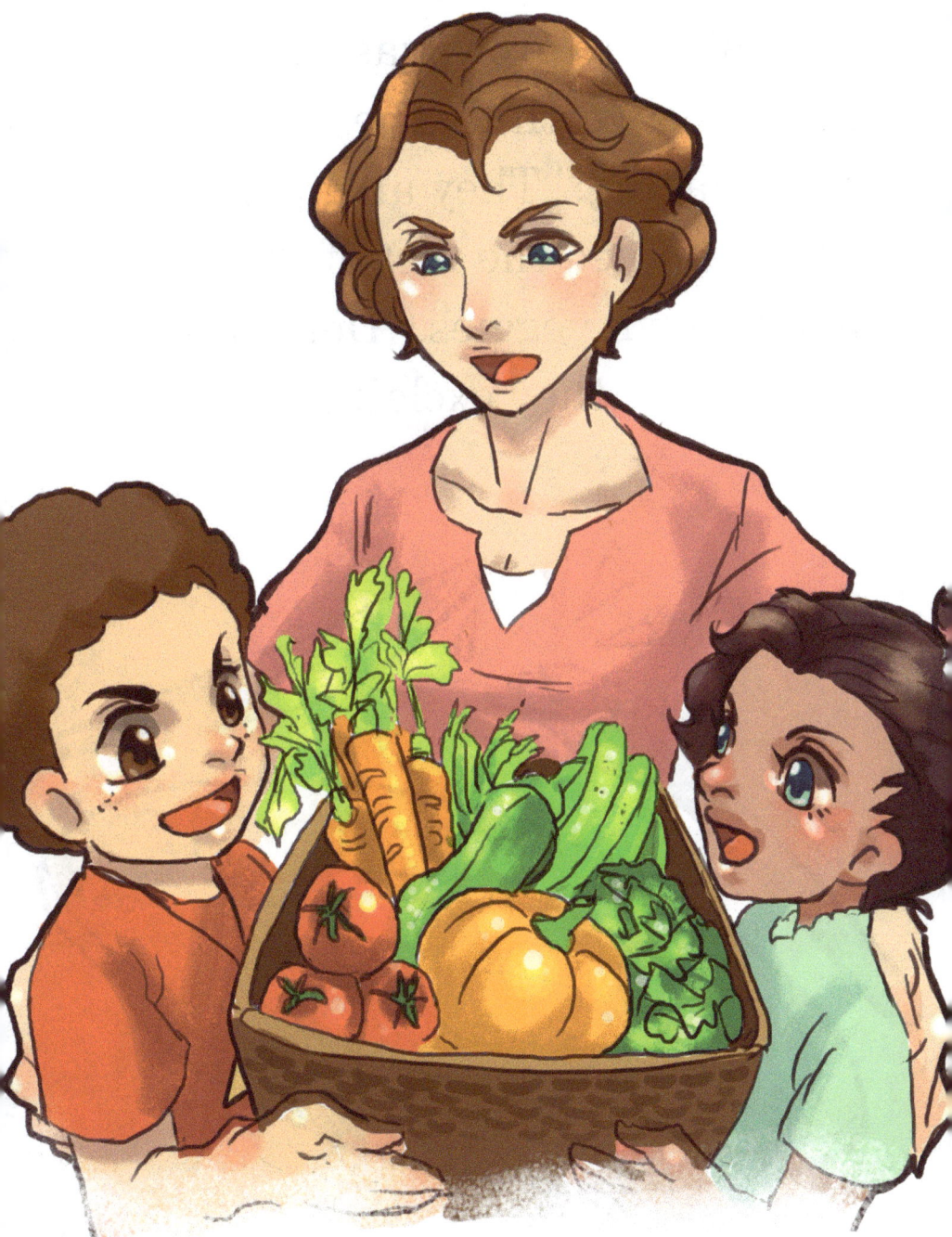

They tasted a green bean. "YUM!"
Healthy Benji said, "Waiting for
vegetables to grow was soooo hard...
but soooo worth it. These vegetables
are amazing!" They all giggled
then sampled the rest of their
homegrown veggies. "Delicious!
What fun!" they exclaimed.

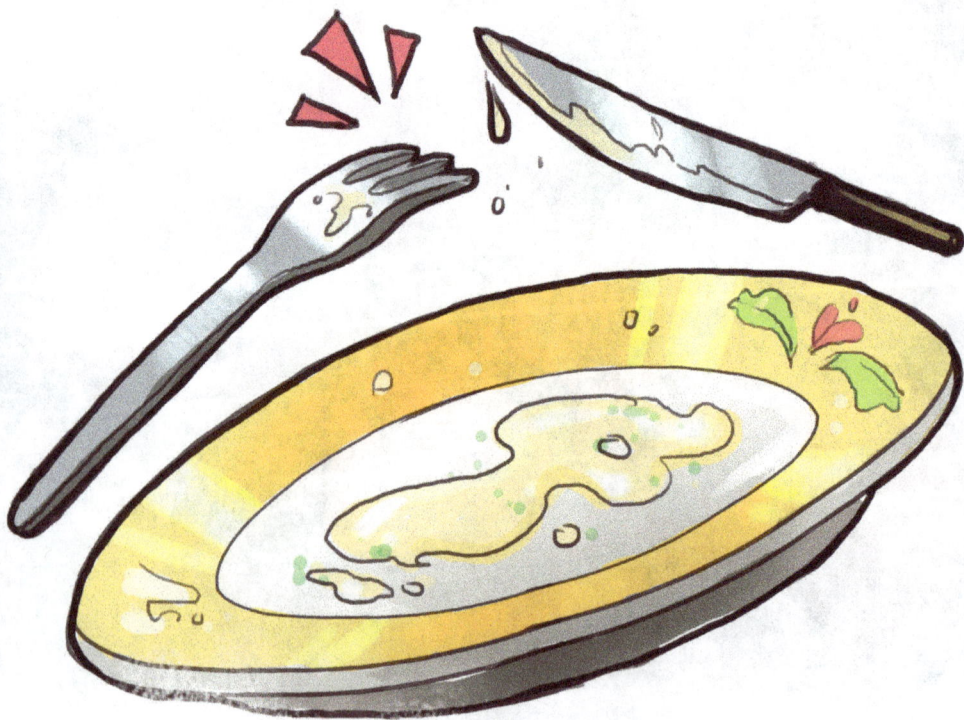

Discussion questions:

Do you have a garden? If not, create one! Grow some vegetables or flowers of your very own.

Make your own bird feeder for the birds in your yard. Watch how they enjoy the bird food!

Make a potato head planter, just like Healthy Benji and Nadia. Decorate your potato and grow your own grass hair!

What kind of vegetables would you like to have in your garden?

What kind of things would you do while you were waiting for your garden to grow? Get some exercise? Make a craft? Feed the squirrels? What kind of activity do you like best?

FACTS ABOUT THE GARDEN

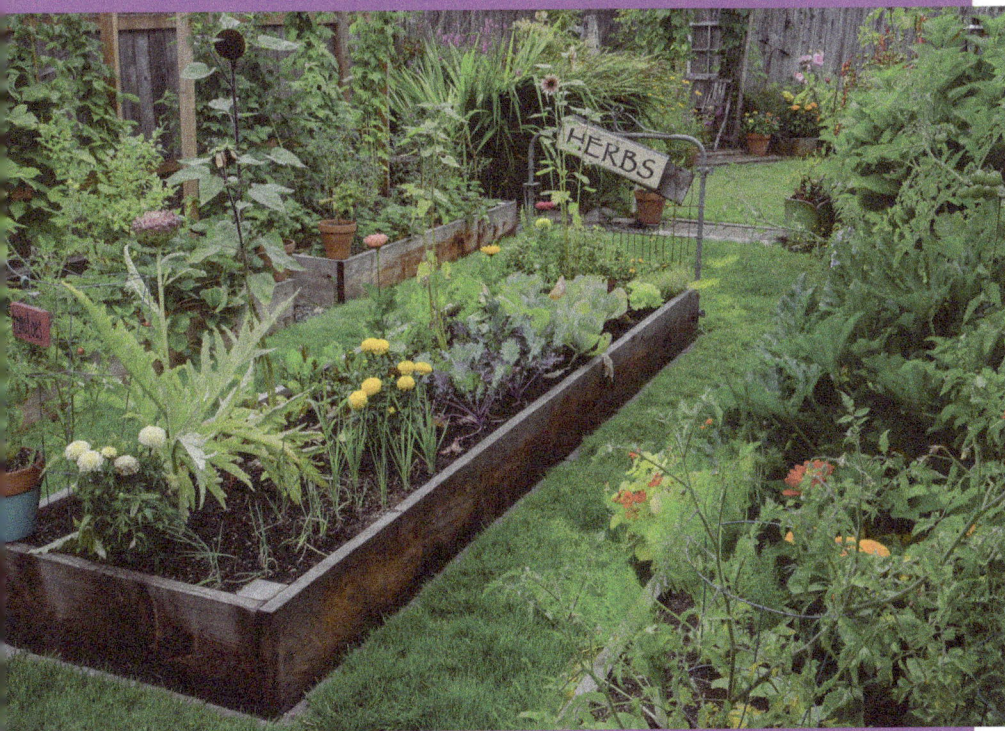

BEST GUIDE TO SUCCESSFUL GARDENING

Great list of friends and foes for ten common vegetables. Best to plant foes and friends on opposite sides of the garden or at least 4 feet away

BEANS	
FRIEND	FOE
Beets	Garlic
Broccoli	Onions
Cabbage	Peppers
Carrots	Sunflowers
Cauliflower	
Celery	
Corn	
Cucumbers	
Eggplant	
Peas	
Potatoes	
Radishes	
Squash	
Strawberries	
Summer	
savory	
Tomatoes	

LETTUCE	
FRIEND	FOE
Asparagus	Broccoli
Beets	
Brussels	
sprouts	
Cabbage	
Carrots	
Corn	
Cucumbers	
Eggplant	
Onions	
Peas	
Potatoes	
Radishes	
Spinach	
Strawberries	
Sunflowers	
Tomatoes	

ONIONS	
FRIEND	FOE
Beets	Beans
Broccoli	Peas
Cabbage	Sage
Carrots	
Lettuce	
Peppers	
Potatoes	
Spinach	
Tomatoes	

CUCUMBERS	
FRIEND	FOE
Beans	Aromatic
Cabbage	herbs
Cauliflower	Melons
Corn	Potatoes
Lettuce	
Peas	
Radishes	
Sunflowers	

CARROTS	
FRIEND	FOE
Beans	Anise
Lettuce	Dill
Onions	Parsley
Peas	
Radishes	
Rosemary	
Sage	
Tomatoes	

CORN	
FRIEND	FOE
Beans	Tomatoes
Cucumbers	
Lettuce	
Melons	
Peas	
Potatoes	
Squash	
Sunflowers	

PEPPERS	
FRIEND	FOE
Basil	Beans
Coriander	Kohlrabi
Onions	
Spinach	
Tomatoes	

RADISHES	
FRIEND	FOE
Basil	Beans
Coriander	Kohlrabi
Onions	
Spinach	
Tomatoes	

CABBAGE	
FRIEND	FOE
Beans	Broccoli
Celery	Cauliflower
Cucumbers	Strawberries
Dill	Tomatoes
Kale	
Lettuce	
Onions	
Potatoes	
Sage	
Spinach	
Thyme	

TOMATOES	
FRIEND	FOE
Asparagus	Broccoli
Basil	Brussels
Beans	sprouts
Borage	Cabbage
Carrots	Cauliflower
Celery	Corn
Dill	Kale
Lettuce	Potatoes
Melons	
Onions	
Parsley	
Peppers	
Radishes	
Spinach	
Thyme	

http://www.almanac.com/content/plant-companions-list-ten-common-vegetables

TIPS FOR YOUR VEGETABLE GARDEN

One of the keys to successful companion planting is observation. Record your plant combinations and the results from year to year, and share this information with other gardening friends. Companionship is just as important for gardeners as it is for gardens.

- Some plants, especially herbs, act as repellents, confusing insects with their strong odors that mask the scent of the intended host plants.

- Dill and basil planted among tomatoes protect the tomatoes from hornworms, and sage scattered about the cabbage patch reduces injury from cabbage moths.

- Marigolds are as good as gold when grown with just about any garden plant, repelling beetles, nematodes, and even animal pests.

- Some companions act as trap plants, luring insects to themselves. Nasturtiums, for example, are so favored by aphids that the devastating insects will flock to them instead of other plants.

- Carrots, dill, parsley, and parsnip attract garden heroes — praying mantises, ladybugs, and spiders — that dine on insect pests.

- Much of companion planting is common sense: Lettuce, radishes, and other quick-growing plants sown between hills of melons or winter squash will mature and be harvested long before these vines need more leg room.

- Leafy greens like spinach and Swiss chard grown in the shadow of corn

- Sunflowers appreciate the dapple shade that corn casts and, since their roots occupy different levels in the soil, don't compete for water and nutrients.

Strange Pairings

Sometimes plants may be helpful to one another only at a certain stage of their growth. The number and ratio of different plants growing together is often a factor in their compatibility, and sometimes plants make good companions for no apparent reason.

- You would assume that keeping a garden weed-free would be a good thing, but this is not always the case. Certain weeds pull nutrients from deep in the soil and bring them close to the surface. When the weeds die and decompose, nutrients become available in the surface soil and are more easily accessed by shallow-rooted plants.

- Perhaps one of the most intriguing examples of strange garden bedfellows is the relationship between the weed stinging nettle and several vegetable varieties. For reasons that are unclear, plants grown in the presence of stinging nettle display exceptional vigor and resist spoiling.

CUCUMBERS

Preferred Growing Conditions

Of course, cucumbers need lots of sun—full sun, in fact. Vegetable gardens should have 6-8 hours a full sunlight a day. Cucumbers, also, like warm weather. If you have a limited growing season, start cucumber seedlings indoors early, so you'll be ready to plant when the warm weather arrives. But wait till soil temperatures have reached 70 degrees Fahrenheit. Even light frosts will kill these plants.

Cucumbers like soil rich in organic matter, well drained, and around a neutral pH (around 6.5). These all really go hand in hand, anyway. Just add some compost to your soil or your planter, and it should take care of the three soil preferences of cucumbers. Cucumber plants are flexible with the pH level. So, they'll do great as long as the pH level is around 6.5.

Really though, don't stress about soil conditions. Cucumbers are hearty plants and easy to grow. Just make sure they have full sunlight and soil is rich in organic matter.

Remember, mulch helps soil retain moisture. When vegetables like full sun, soil tends to dry out quickly. Mulch, also, will keep the cucumbers off the soil away from pests and clean.

How to Plant Cucumbers

Cucumbers can be planted in containers, rows, hills, or raised beds. Be warned: one plant produces a lot of cucumbers.

And, some plants can produce all summer long. So, think about spacing out plantings to harvest all season.

Containers

Cucumbers grow as bushes or vines. Bush varieties grow well in containers. Refer to the variety list above for types of cucumbers suitable for containers and planters. Vine cucumbers will need a trellis, and there's more space for those in a garden out in the yard.

Rows

You can plant rows of cucumbers once soil temperature is 70 degrees Fahrenheit. Space rows 6 ½ feet apart, and plants should have about 2 ½ feet between them. But check your variety, if growing a smaller cucumber plant, you may be able to add more plants in a smaller space. There are some varieties that only need 8-10 inches between the plants.

TOMATOES

There are two basic kinds of tomatoes: Determinate and Indeterminate.

- Determinate tomatoes produce the fruit all at once. These are typically bush tomatoes, and make the best tomatoes for container gardening. Since all the tomatoes are ripe within a short period of time, these are great plant choices if you plan to can or have a short tomato growing season.

- Indeterminate tomatoes grow on a vine. They will produce all season until the first frost.

Preferred Growing Conditions

Tomatoes love sun, and lots of it. Determinate or bush tomato plants work best for tomato container gardening. Soil should be rich in organic matter. Compost works best mixed in with the soil, and is a great organic fertilizer. Tomatoes tend to do well in soil that is a little acidic. Get a soil pH tester if you are unsure of your soil's pH level.

Mulch will be important around tomato plants. Since tomato plants prefer full sun, the soil will dry out. Mulch will help retain moisture in the soil.

How to Plant Tomatoes

Space out tomato plants 13 – 17 inches apart. Really just follow the planting instructions with the variety you choose. It will all depend on the variety of tomato you grow. You just want to make sure they will have enough room to grow and the roots not compete with each other. You can plant tomato seedlings after the last frost. Seeds can be started just before the last frost.

Keep in mind tomatoes do well in raised beds. If you are not planting in a raised bed, raise your tomato rows about six inches in the garden. Rows should be 4-5 feet apart. But, don't forget that determinate tomato varieties grow well in containers, too!

Companion Plants for Tomatoes

Growing these companion plants around tomatoes will be helpful: basil, chives, oregano, parsley, onions, carrots, asparagus, marigolds, celery, and geraniums.

Some plants actually are bad to the health of tomato plants. Avoid these plants around tomatoes: black walnut, corn, cabbage, potatoes, kale, and rosemary.

Maintaining Your Tomato Plants

Not sure what to do in the meantime? You will most likely need to stake your tomatoes. Again, depends on the variety. Bush tomatoes may need to be staked or caged for support. But, indeterminate tomatoes, or vine tomatoes, will definitely need support since they continue to grow all season. A trellis works nicely with vine tomatoes or a tomato cage.

Should you prune tomatoes? Depends on who you ask! Suckers, or side shoots, grow in the "v" of the stem and branch.

You can pinch them off or leave them. Leaving the suckers on produces more tomatoes. But these will be smaller tomatoes. If you have a large tomato plant, like the indeterminate, you might want to prune the side shoots here and there. But don't go hog wild, you want these plants to produce.

When to Use Organic Fertilizer

It's a good idea to use organic fertilizer in your garden, and avoid the chemicals around your food. Typically, tomatoes are fertilized every 3-4 weeks, with the first fertilization at planting. The next time you're ready to fertilize should be about the time the plant is bearing small tomatoes. Some determinate varieties will only be fertilized two times, since they produce tomatoes all at once.

You can also find products at nurseries, like Tomato Thrive, a microbial growth promoter, that help tomato plants absorb nutrients from the soil. This makes your fertilizer absorb better, too.

When to Harvest Tomatoes

Tomatoes take 50-80 days to harvest. Just pick them when they have turned their full color. You can pick them early and let them ripen in the windowsill. But, the best tomato flavor is one that has ripened on the vine.

Tomato Pests and Diseases

Keep an eye out for tomato hornworms. They are the large, beautiful green worms that blend nicely with the stems.

http://www.almanac.com/content/plant-companions-list-ten-common-vegetables

DID YOU KNOW?

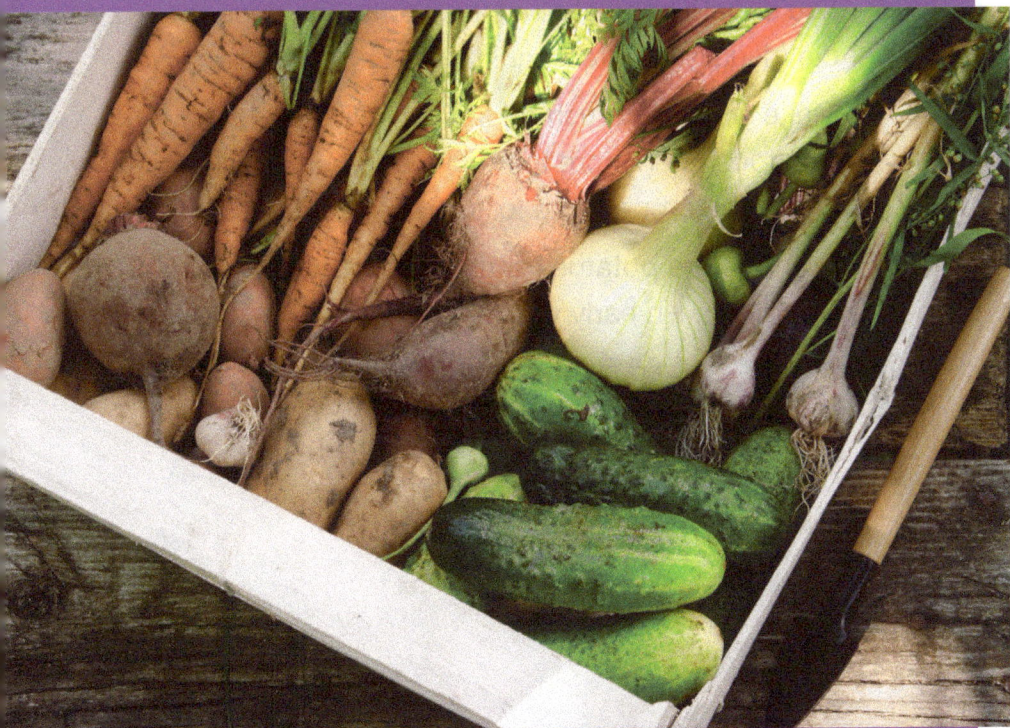

DID YOU KNOW...?

- Potato is a vegetable that should be planted in full sun, sandy soil with acidic soil

- Plant about two weeks after the last winter frost

- Spread and mix in rotted manure or organic compost in the bottom of the trench before planting Dig potatoes on a dry day. Dig up gently, being careful not to puncture the tubers. The soil should not be compact, so digging should be easy.

- New potatoes will be ready for harvest after 10 weeks, usually in early July.

- You should harvest all of your potatoes once the vines die (usually by late August), or the potatoes may rot.

- Make sure you brush off any soil clinging to the potatoes, then store them in a cool, dry, dark place. The ideal temperature for storage is 35 to 40°F.

- Do not store potatoes with apples; their ethylene' Irish Cobbler' is an early variety.

- 'Viking' is a red skinned potato, regular season variety.

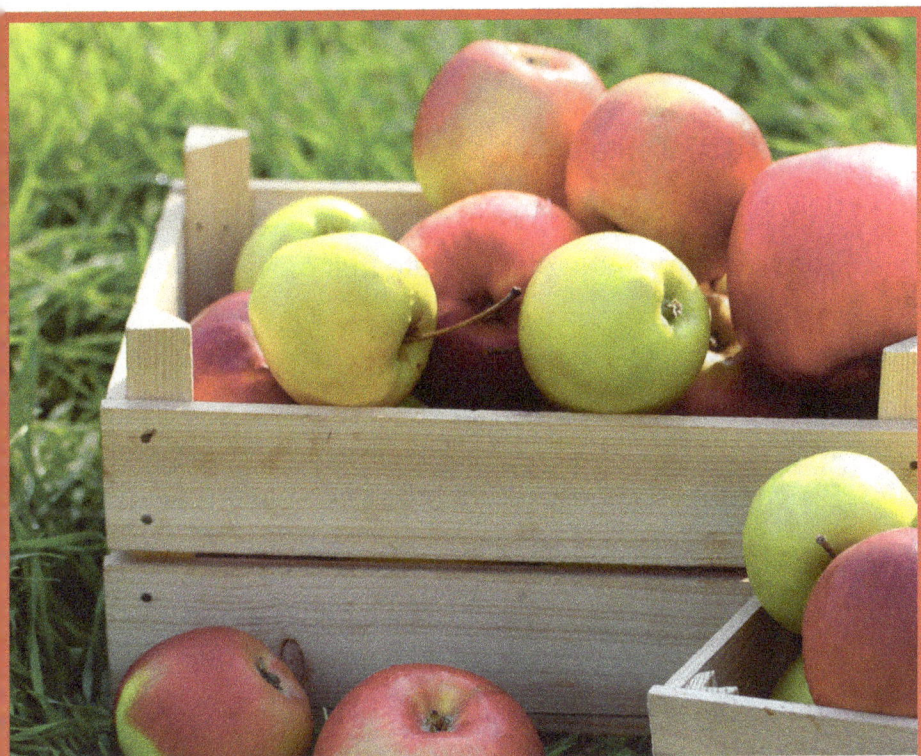

DID YOU KNOW...?

- Don't peel your apple! Most of the fiber and many antioxidants are found in the apple peel.

- The largest apple picked weighed three pounds.

- Red Delicious, Golden Delicious, Granny Smith, Gala and Fuji are the top five apples eaten in the United States.

- Apples are a member of the rose family, along with pears, peaches, plums and cherries.

- One apple has five grams of fiber.

- Apples are fat, sodium, and cholesterol free.

DID YOU KNOW...?

- America's favorite muffin is blueberry.
- July is national blueberry month.
- The blueberry is the official state fruit of New Jersey.
- There are over 200 species of raspberries.
- Raspberries can be red, black, yellow, or purple.
- Blackberries are high in Vitamin C and fiber.
- Blackberries are helpful in the treatment of stomach problems.

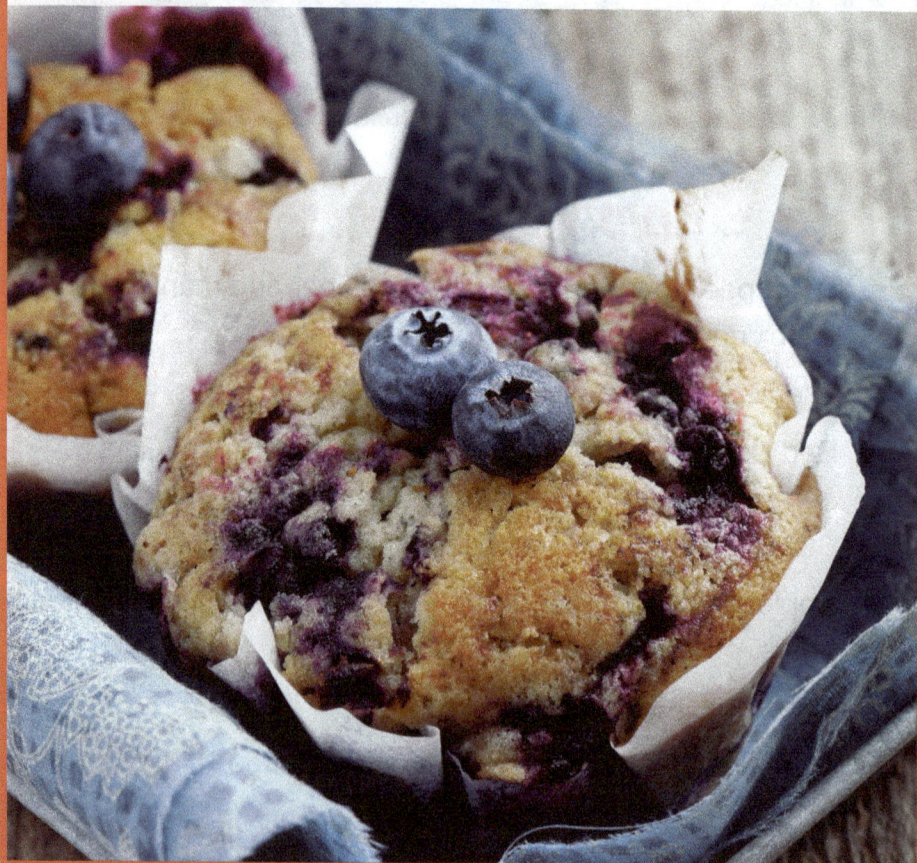

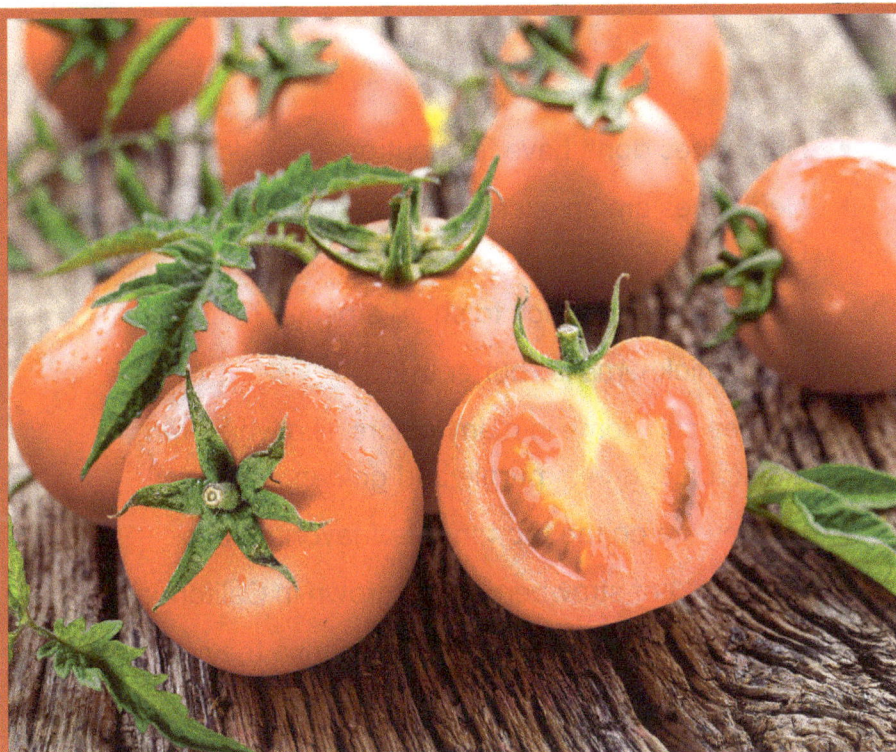

DID YOU KNOW...?

- There are at least 25,000 varieties of tomatoes.
- Tomatoes have been called "wolf peach," "a plump thing with a navel," and "the apple of love."
- Mushrooms do not need sunshine to grow and thrive.
- The pepper is actually a fruit, not a vegetable.
- Peppers come in many colors, including green, yellow, orange, red, brown, and purple.

DID YOU KNOW...?

- Nectarines don't have fuzz but peaches do.
- Nectarines are an excellent source of vitamins A and C.
- In China, it's bad luck to share a pear.
- Pear's nickname is "butter fruit."
- Grapes can come in many colors, like white, red, black, blue, green, purple and golden.
- Grapes are on the top ten list of favorite fruits.
- Over 80% of strawberries are grown in California.
- Strawberries are hand-picked because they are so fragile.

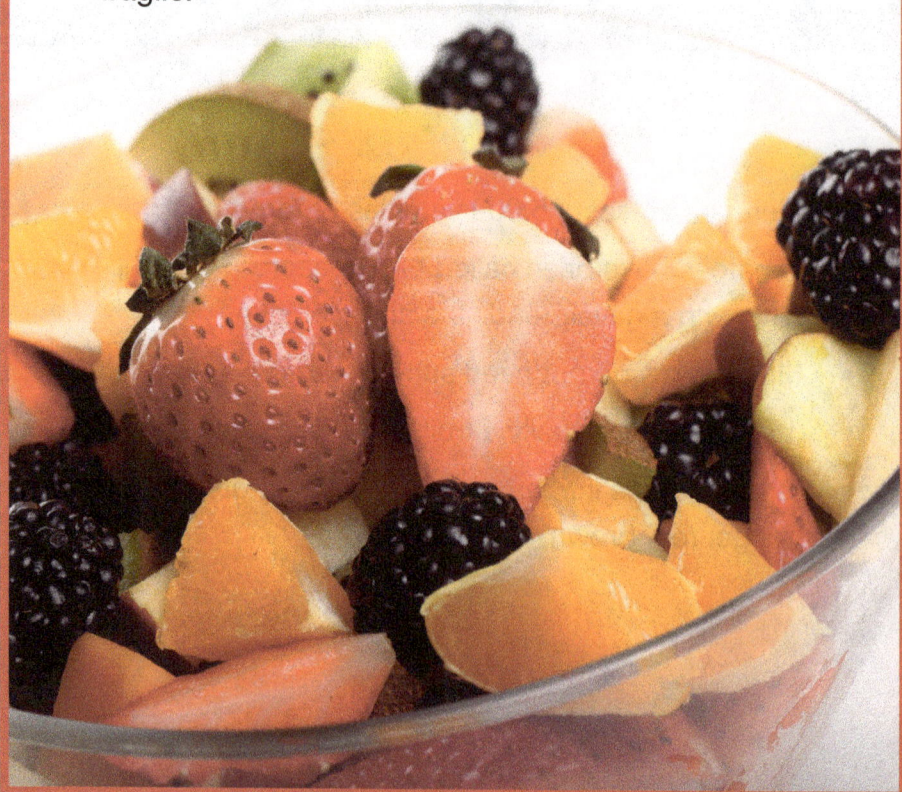

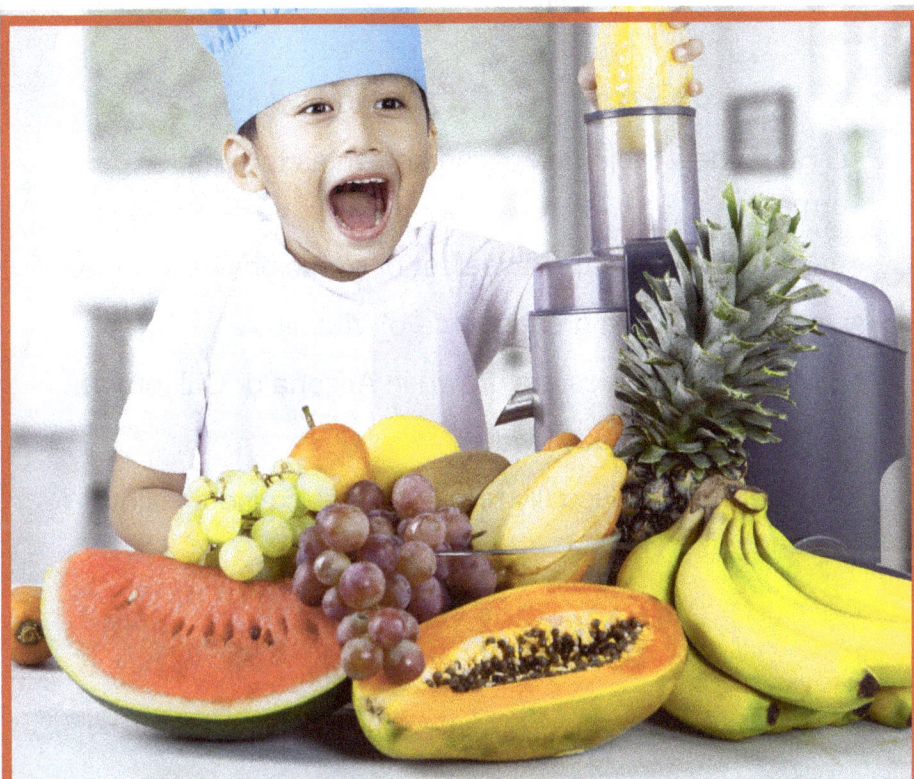

DID YOU KNOW...?

- Bananas, apples, and watermelons float in water.
- The average American eats 27 pounds of bananas each year!
- An individual banana is called a finger. A bunch of bananas is called a hand.
- Bananas are a good source of vitamin B6, which your brain needs to function properly and make you wise.
- Mangoes are related to cashews and pistachios
- The mango is a symbol of love in India.

DID YOU KNOW...?

- Honeydew melons are also known as temptation melons.

- Honeydews are the sweetest of all melons when ripe.

- Cantaloupe is a great source of Vitamin A.

- Most cantaloupes are grown in Arizona or California.

- Watermelon is 92% water.

- Watermelon is usually red, but there is also a yellow variety.

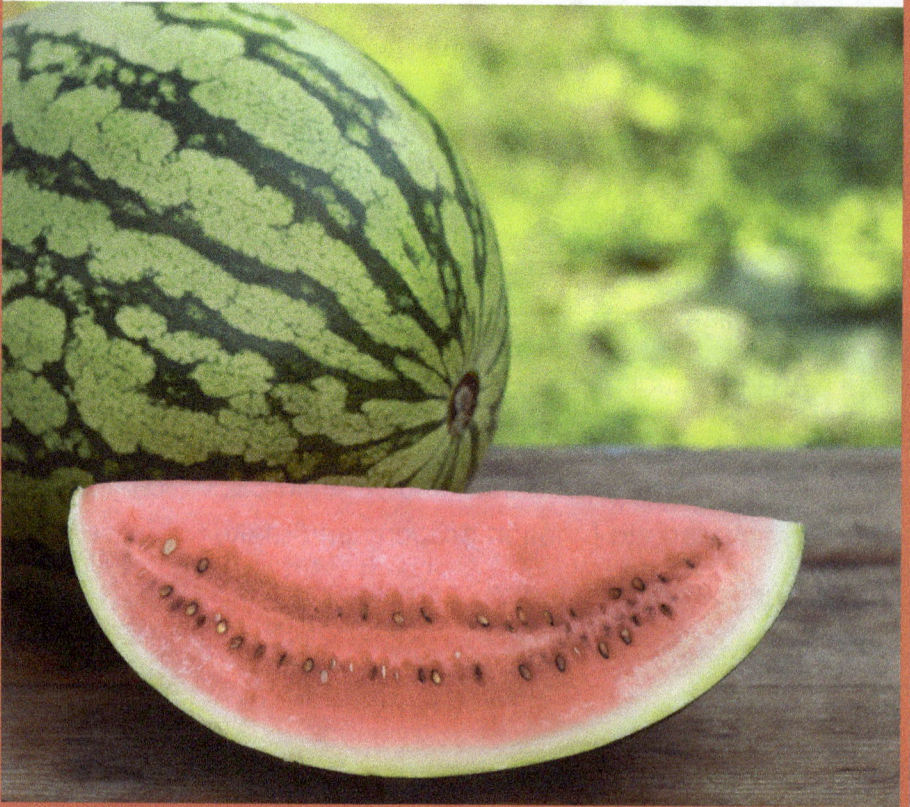

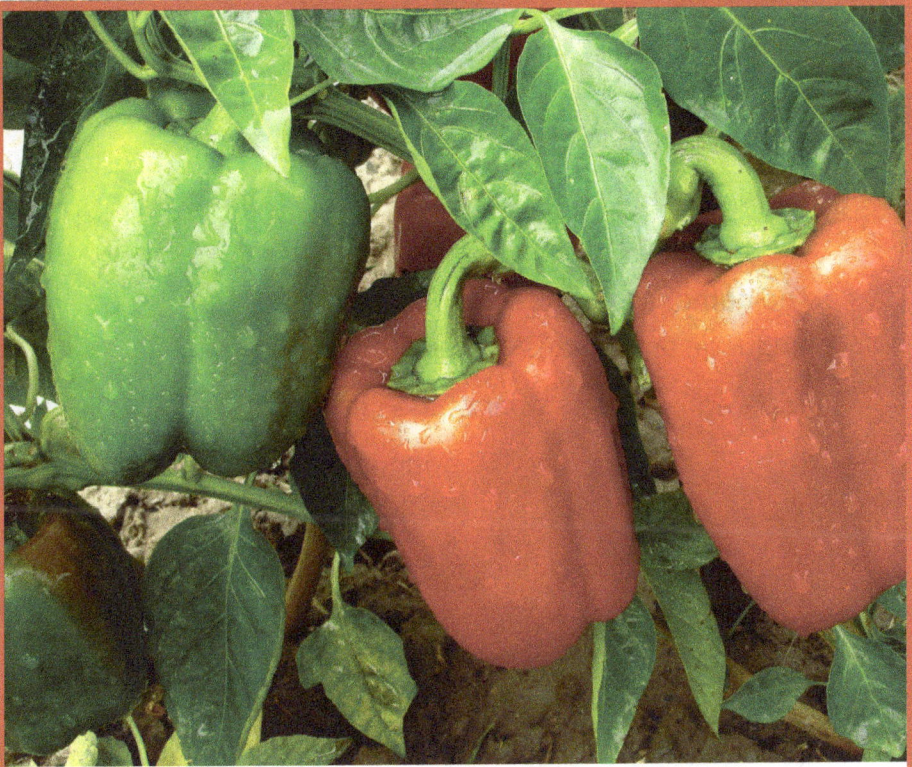

DID YOU KNOW...?

- Peppers are actually fruits that form on the plant after it flowers.
- Peppers can be green, red, yellow, and orange.
- Sometimes peppers can even be white, purple, blue, and brown, depending on when they are harvested.
- Tomatoes are actually a fruit.
- Tomato season is from June to November.
- Onion can help remove warts.
- Onions can soothe an insect bite.

DID YOU KNOW...?

- A zucchini has more potassium than a banana.

- The word zucchini comes from "zucca" the Italian word for squash.

- The name, asparagus, comes from the Greek language and means "sprout" or "shoot."

- Asparagus is a member of the Lily family.

- In 1974, a man grew 370 pounds of potatoes on one plant.

- Buds on potatoes are called "eyes."

- The world's largest potato chip measured 23 feet x 14.5 feet.

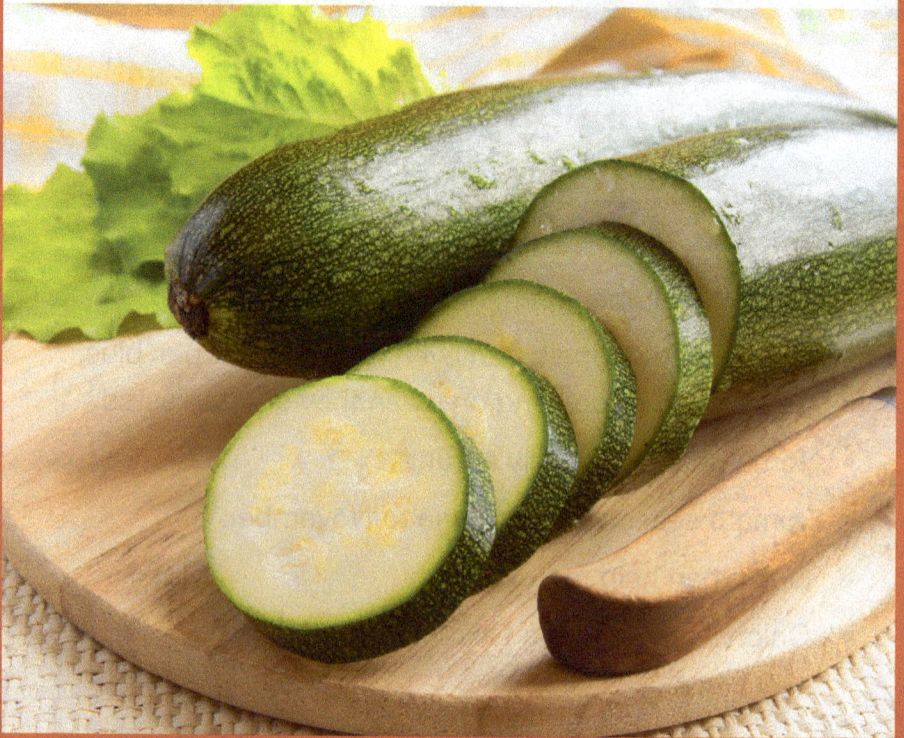

DID YOU KNOW...?

- The average person in the United States eats four and one half pounds of broccoli each year.

- Broccoli got its name from the Latin word bracchium, which means strong arm or branch. They look like little trees!

- California and Arizona produced 100% of the national total.

- Cabbage can be purple or green.

- Cabbage can improve digestion.

- The snow pea is also called the "China mangetout."

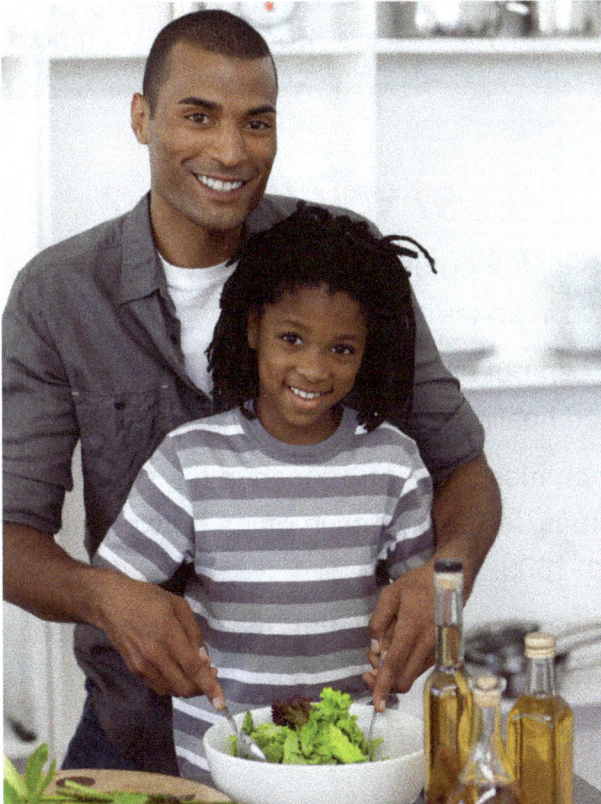

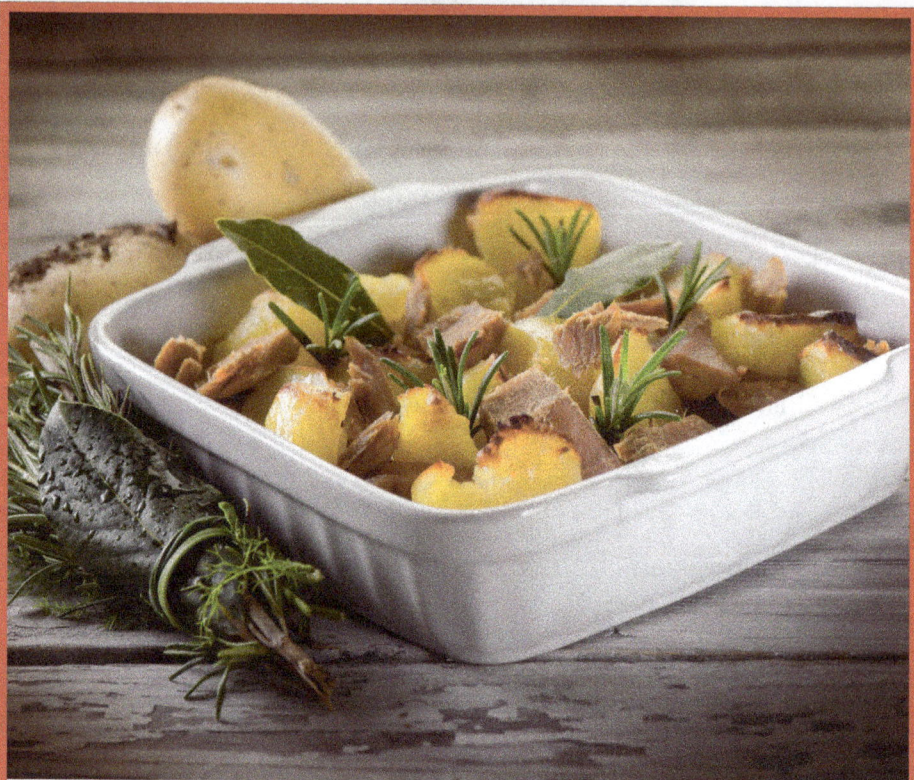

DID YOU KNOW...?

- In 1995, the potato was the first vegetable to be grown in space.

- You can put slices of raw potato on broken bones to speed healing.

- French fries were introduced in the states when Thomas Jefferson was in office between the years of 1801-1809.

- Eating potatoes with other foods can prevent indigestion.

- Potato chips were invented in 1853.

DID YOU KNOW...?

- The Aztecs made what may be the first salsa – tomatoes prepared with peppers, corn, and salt.

- China is the world's largest producer of tomatoes.

- The leaves of a tomato plant are poisonous.

- Green beans can actually be green, yellow, purple, or speckled in those colors.

- Green beans vary in size, but the average length is about 4 inches.

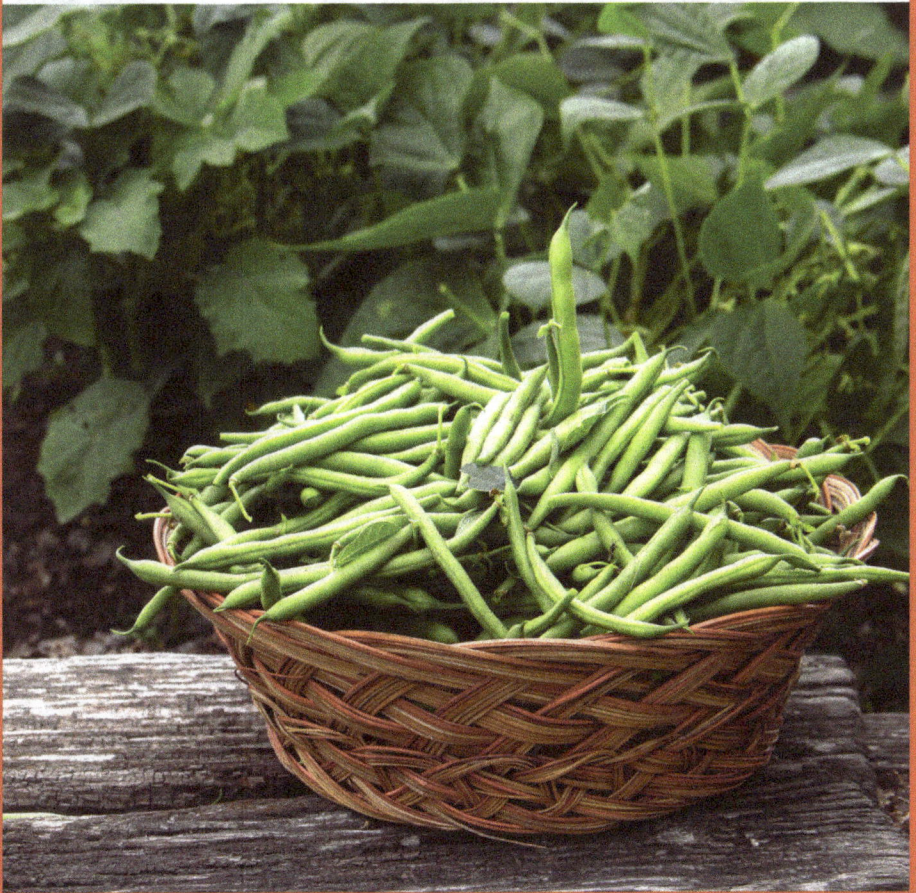

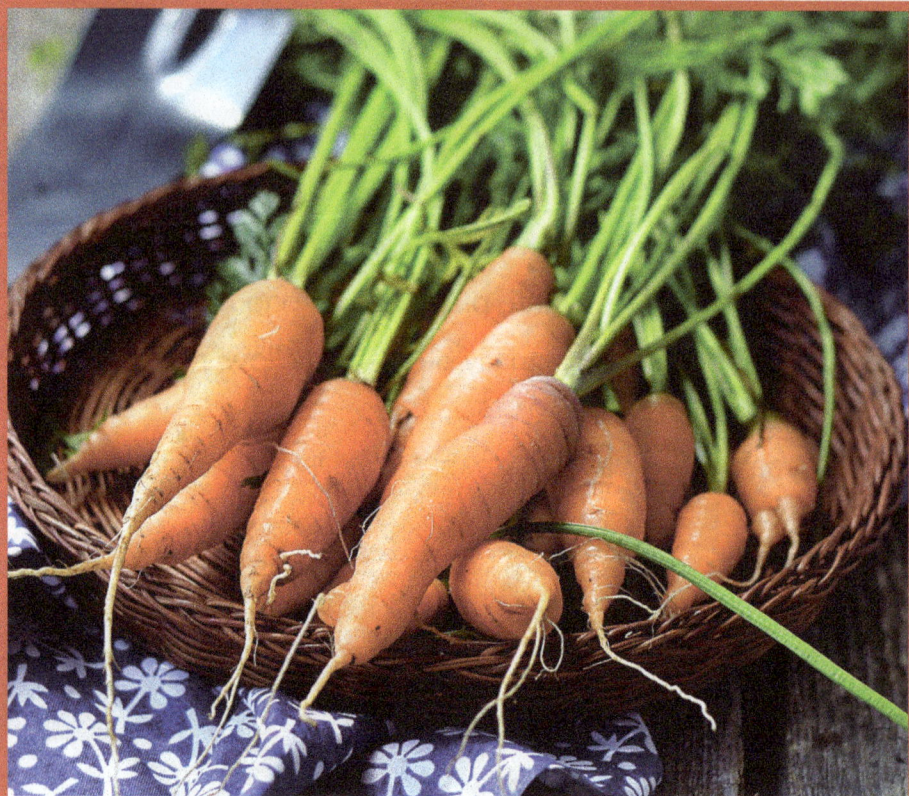

DID YOU KNOW...?

- Lima beans are rich source of antioxidants, vitamins, minerals, and fiber.

- Carrots help improve eyesight, especially at night.

- Carrots help keep your skin and hair healthy.

- Carrots have the highest beta-carotene of any vegetable.

- Holtville, California dubs itself "The Carrot Capital of the World."

- The largest cabbage on record weighed 123 pounds.

- A cabbage can grow in three months time.

DID YOU KNOW...?

- Bok choy is also known as Chinese cabbage.

- Bok choy is very nutritious, it's high in Vitamin A, Vitamin C, potassium and calcium.

- Tofu acts like a sponge and has the miraculous ability to soak up any flavor that is added to it.

- Tofu is also known as soybean curd.

- Green onions are also known as scallions.

- On a green onion, the white bulb and the green stalk are both edible.

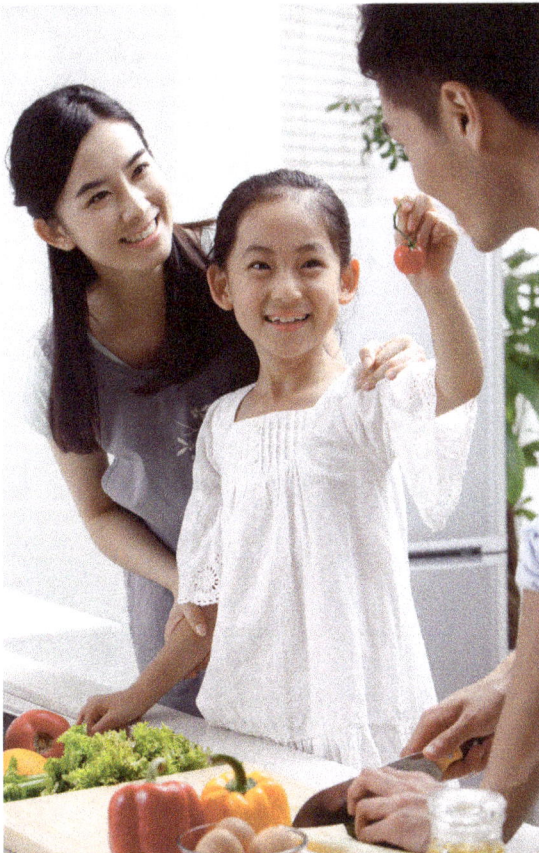

* 9 7 8 0 9 9 1 0 3 6 1 3 4 *